In this book you will discover the most effective and healthy fat-loss program ever presented.

In the following pages...

You will realize that it's your percentage of body fat—not your body weight— that defines your health and wellness.

You will develop the skills to measure and manage your body fat— helping you to live a longer and healthier life.

You will learn how to cook healthy, low-fat meals— with less time and effort than you ever imagined.

You will follow a simple and effective exercise program that promises to achieve lasting results —no matter what your fitness level!

You will look and feel better than you ever imagined...

...so read on and get ready to

Combat Fat!

Combat Fat!

Andrew Flach

with
RoseMarie Alfieri
Stew Smith
James Villepigue

AND

M. Laurel Cutlip, LN, RD

Photographs by Peter Field Peck
Cartoons by Randy Glasbergen

Hatherleigh Press

Combat Fat!
A Hatherleigh Press Book

Text and photos © Copyright 2002 The Hatherleigh Company, Ltd.
All rights reserved. No part of this book maybe reproduced in any form or by any means,
electronic or mechanical, including photocopying, recording, or by any information
storage and retrieval system, without permission in writing from the publisher.

Hatherleigh Press
An Affiliate of W.W. Norton and Company, Inc.
5-22 46th Avenue, Suite 200
Long Island CIty, NY 11101
Toll Free 1-800-528-2550
Visit our websites getfitnow.com and hatherleighpress.com

DISCLAIMER:
Before beginning any diet and exercise program, consult your physician. The authors and the publisher disclaim any lia-
bility, personal or professional, resulting from the application or misapplication of any of the information in this publication.

Combat Fat! books are available for bulk purchase, special promotions and
premiums. For more information on reselling and special purchase opportunities, please call us
at 1-800-528-2550 and ask for the Special Sales Manager.

LIBRARY OF CONGRESS CATALOGING AND PUBLICATION DATA TO COME
ISBN: 1-57826-089-2

Interior Layout and Design Angel Harleycat

Cover Design by Angel Harleycat

10 9 8 7 6 5 4 3 2 1
Printed in Canada on acid-free paper.

Table of Contents

Acknowledgements

We are grateful to the following:

The wonderful publishing, editorial, and production staff at Hatherleigh Press, including Kevin Moran, Fatema Tarzi, Jenny Noguerol, and Peter Peck for their incredible support throughout this project.

The diligent W.W. Norton Company sales and management team including Dosier Hammond, Bill Rusin, Stephen King, John DiBello, and Soo Jin Oh for their encouragement and extraordinary effort.

To Matt Chalek of Accu-Measure, LLC, whose products help men and women live healthier lives.

Dedication

This book is dedicated to everyone who wants to be the healthiest they can be!

Preface
by Andrew Flach

When I was told that I was carrying 50 pounds of fat on my body I was shocked! At 6'4" and 200 pounds, I thought I was in okay shape. Sure I didn't eat the best, being a busy person, but that was never a problem. As a kid I was always skinny as a string bean. No matter what I ate, I never put on the pounds.

My Life at a Crossroads

Now there I was, age 39, on the verge of obesity. Not for a lack of willpower but a lack of knowledge. I just didn't know how much fat I had. I didn't know how to measure it. I thought my weight was okay. My clothes still fit (although some of my pants were getting a bit tight in the waist). In the mirror I looked o.k. None of my friends commented that I was looking heavy.

But the fat was there all right. And the calipers proved it. A visit to the doctor for a routine medical reported that my cholesterol was too high—raising a red flag on my blood test. On the eve of my fortieth birthday I was in sore need of a change.

Oh, one other thing I should mention. My career to date was that of a writer and publisher—of all things—fitness and health books! How then could I purvey information for men and women to take better care of themselves, when I myself was not living up to the standard? What excuse could I possibly have?

Well, for one, I am human. Human beings are not perfect. Never will be. That's just part of the package. Sure we aspire, dream, hope, and achieve—but, too, we also procrastinate, get discouraged and lazy, and fail. That's just the way it is. But we can pick up the pieces and start over, as many times as we can, each time getting better and better. Our lives should be lived in a constant cycle of self-improvement. It was time again for me to rethink and revisit my personal health and fitness goals.

Fortunately, I had working in my office a gentleman named James Villepique. I had hired James earlier that year to help me with my publishing business and website, Getfitnow.com. In fact, James found us through one of our books and wrote to me directly asking for a job. He came with a long list of experiences in the fitness profession: a personal trainer, a writer, an inventor, and a martial arts expert.

I asked James to help me put together a personal fitness and exercise plan that I could follow. I started immediately. Four days a week of weight training combined with two days of intensive cardiovascular training on the treadmill.

From my diet, I was to cut out my favorite bachelor foods—pizza, lo mein, cheeseburgers—and start eating more sensibly. Chicken breast, vegetables, salad, fruits, turkey burgers. Nothing complicated, just sensible.

I learned another thing from James—that it was essential for me to eat breakfast. I was a big time breakfast skipper (and who isn't?). I learned that of all meals of the day breakfast is perhaps the most important one. It gives you the energy to carry forth with vigor and vitality. It starts a metabolism cycle that continues throughout the day. James also recommended that I have a mid-morning and mid-afternoon snack. Nothing too much, but something healthy to maintain my energy level.

I exercised after work each day, committing about one-hour worth of my

x

free time to my effort. I must admit that although I was in "decent" shape (or so I thought) the workouts were painful. Not pain as in muscle pain. But pain as in psychic pain. It really hurt to think that I had slipped so far down the ladder of health and fitness! I had always thought of myself as a relatively fit person, but the truth lay in the numbers. I couldn't curl more than 15 pounds, basic lunges were a test, and my chest press was dismal. But I found weights that I could use and kept with the program until I was able to progress to heavier weights.

And that's one thing that's very exciting and real—the human body responds positively to physical training. At any age and any fitness level you will realize gains. Gains in strength from weight training, gains in flexibility from stretching, gains in endurance from cardiovascular exercise.

So I stayed with it. And I was transformed—physically. I developed lean muscle. I shed excess fat. I felt better than I had in years. And my transformation led to the idea that we should put a book together to share the good news to others. Such was the birth of Combat Fat!

America at a Crossroads

In the months since then, my research has uncovered a real health crisis in the United States—the increasing trend of obesity in both teenagers and adults. The numbers were unbelievable—but true. The rate of growth— exponential. I recognized that there was a real need to create a book that would help all of us take more responsibility for our health and well being. Our own survival, the very survival of our nation depends on it.

The United States, the most prosperous nation on earth, is getting fat. And fat America is killing itself. More than 300,000 premature deaths per year are attributable to obesity and lack of physical activity! That's second only to tobacco-related deaths!

The diseases relating to obesity include diabetes, high blood pressure, heart disease, and cancer. I have known people who have died from their obesity or from complications related to their obesity. These people could have been helped, or could have helped themselves, had they known what to do.

So it is my mission—our mission—to educate millions of Americans about the dangers of being too fat and how they can take command of their lives and their health by eating intelligently and exercising regularly.

We have put together a simple yet effective plan, which can be adapted to fit anyone's lifestyle and finances. Fitness is not just for the fit. Nor is it just for the rich. Fitness is a right for everyone. You have a right to be fit! We will give you the proper knowledge and right tools to do the job. All we ask is that you try.

Recognize that it may not be easy at the beginning. But try nonetheless. Stick with it. When it gets tough, reach out for support. We are there for you. "No man is an island," said a famous poet a long time ago. We are all in this together. We have all been through this before. We will all achieve success and victory!

Mission: Impossible? No! Mission: Possible!

When I was a kid my favorite television show was *Mission: Impossible*. I always loved the very beginning of the show, when Mr. Phelps received his orders via the self-destructing tape recorder: "Good Morning Mr. Phelps...etc."

Phelps then went on to select the team members who would participate in the current assignment. Each member of the Impossible Mission team possessed a unique talent which contributed to the success of the job: Barney, the wiz at electronics. Willy, the strong man; Cinnamon, the alluring seductress; and so on.

Well when it came time to write this book, I thought of the *Mission: Impossible* analogy. So here it goes—

You walk to the local grocery store and pick up a box of coffeecake. You carry the box to a remote part of the aisle and open it. Inside is a small cassette recorder. You push the "play button".

> *Good Morning Mr./Ms._____.*
> *Excess fat is the enemy. Too much fat can lead*
> *to diabetes, heart disease, and other illnesses.*
> *Too much fat can lead to premature death. We*
> *already have the knowledge to take command of*
> *the situation. You will discover that fat can be*
> *measured, its growth can be halted, its presence*
> *can be reduced. Your mission, should you choose*
> *to accept it (and we know you can!), is to lower*
> *your caloric intake, exercise regularly each week,*
> *reduce your consumption of sugar and fatty*
> *foods, and aspire to live a healthy, vibrant life!*
> *If you or any member of your Combat Fat!*
> *team should ever have a setback, we will be*
> *there for you! This coffeecake will self-destruct*
> *in 5 seconds.*
>
> *Good luck!*

You immediately drop the box of coffeecake into a nearby trash can where, with a muffled "bang," the cake explodes.

Now we come to the part of the show where we meet the other members of the Combat Fat! Team:

RoseMarie Alfieri: Certified fitness professional and experienced journalist. Expert in health education, group exercise, and personal training.

Laurie Cutlip: Registered Dietitian. Served her country in the United States Navy. Now a full-time nutritionist and health professional. Loves to share healthy recipes.

Stewart Smith: Former Navy SEAL, now full-time fitness professional. Understands how to train men and women of all fitness levels. Cross training a specialty. Makes a hobby of writing workout plans.

James Villepique: Certified fitness professional and inventor. Specializes in body sculpting and weight training techniques. Karate expert.

And of, course, there's me.

There you have it—The Combat Fat! Team. Trained. Educated. Dedicated. Committed to helping you succeed in your mission!

Good luck and best wishes for a long and healthy life.

Andrew Flach

1
America's
Health Crisis

This is the chapter where we scare you lean. At least that's the goal. Let's face it—the evidence is as plain as the nose on your face. Too much fat on your body is bad. Too little physical activity is bad. You are going to have to adjust your eating habits and you are going to have to start an exercise program. Otherwise, you might get sick—very sick—and you just might die. That would be a tragedy for all of those who love you as a friend, a parent, a child, or a spouse.

Too much fat and too little exercise can lead to diabetes, high blood pressure, and cardiovascular disease. There is no excuse not to do something about it. You can reduce your body fat and caloric intake by eating healthy, well-balanced meals. You can increase your physical activity by exercising, jogging, walking, gardening, or doing any number of active things. You can substantially improve your health and the quality of your life!

Bottom line: know the risks you face and take positive action to Combat Fat!

OBESITY and PHYSICAL INACTIVITY account for more than 300,000 premature deaths each and every year.

This staggering number is second only to tobacco-related deaths.

Wake up America—it's time to Combat Fat! For decades we have seen one diet after another hit the bestseller lists and, in the quest to achieve an ideal weight, we have tried them all: high carb and low carb; high protein and shake-based diets. Desperate, many of us have done virtually anything, no matter how strange, how foreign to common sense: for example, we've consumed an inordinate amount of grape-fruits when promised that doing so would shed unwanted pounds. And so we have starved, over-exercised, and pushed ourselves hard all in the hopes of seeing the needle on the scale drop to the left. In fact, an overwhelming majority of us report that we are currently on a diet trying to lose weight. And yet, despite all this effort, all of this work, we Americans are fatter than ever.

The frightening truth is that more than half of all Americans are overweight and 24 percent are considered obese by the government's standards. Between 1998 and 1999, obesity rose six percent, affecting all regions of the country and all demographic groups. These numbers make it clear that Americans are in a body fat crisis. So much so that obesity is now considered to be an epidemic by the government, and public health officials are very concerned. Why? Because if you have too much body fat you are at risk for developing a number of serious chronic diseases such as cardiovascular disease, diabetes, and even cancer.

Dr. Jeffrey Koplan, Director of the Centers for Disease Control and Prevention (CDC), calls the continuing epidemic of obesity, *"a critical public health problem."* According to Koplan, obesity and physical inactivity account for more than 300,000 premature deaths each and every year. This staggering number is second only to tobacco-related deaths.

"As obesity rates continue to grow at epidemic proportions in this country, the net effect will be dramatic increases in related chronic health conditions such as diabetes and cardiovascular disease in the future," warns Koplan.

Just this past year, headlines in major newspapers and various media screamed with the news that the prevalence of diabetes has also reached epidemic proportions in the U.S., with nearly 16 million people suffering from the potentially fatal disease.

Government researchers found that the number of diagnosed diabetes cases increased by 33 percent during the last decade; most disturbing is that it is increasing most dramatically in young adults and in adolescents!

We live increasingly sedentary lives—so many of us spend most of our day behind a computer screen or the wheel of a car and our leisure time in front of the television screen. At the same time we have increased our consumption of HIGHLY CALORIC FAST FOODS and the amount of daily calories we take in.

3

Traditionally, type II or adult-onset diabetes is diagnosed in older adults. The implications of younger people and children suffering from this and other obesity-related diseases are powerful: clearly we must do something to reverse the trend toward fatness.

What has caused the over-fatting of America? There are many theories. Most experts agree that a combination of factors, many resulting from the technological advances of the last 50 years, are to blame. For example we live increasingly sedentary lives—in which so many of us spend most of our day behind a computer screen or the wheel of a car and our leisure time in front of the television screen. Instead of moving our bodies they way they were meant to move, we sit and sit and grow fatter and fatter. In addition, cutbacks in school budgets have led to a decrease in physical education classes, which may account for the large number of children and adolescents who now battle obesity.

At the same time that we have decreased our daily activity, we have increased our consumption of highly caloric fast foods and the amount of daily calories we take in. In earlier times people were so active, naturally, as part of their everyday living that they didn't have to think about getting in enough activity or worry too much about what they ate (and what they ate were natural, healthy foods—not the packaged fast foods so prevalent today). We live in very different times, and we need to adapt to these times in a way that improves, not ruins our health and fitness.

The Surgeon General's Report on Physical Activity and Health

In 1996, the Surgeon General of the United States issued the landmark report on Physical Activity and Health. The report, which was based on a review of several of the best scientific studies, determined that physical activity is essential for maintaining a healthy body composition, and noted that by adopting a more active lifestyle (doing as little as 30 minutes of

4

An Economic Theory to America's Obesity Crisis?

In a recent issue of *The New York Times*, writer Virginia Postrel reviewed a paper published by the National Bureau of Economic Research. *The Long Run Growth of Obesity as a Function of Technological Change* proposed the simple theory that "people haven't changed—they've always liked to eat high-calorie food and generally disliked strenuous exertion—but incentives have."

Nowadays, with most Americans spending their work hours behind a desk, rather than performing manual labor, we have lost a "paid opportunity" to burn excess calories. In the "good old days" we used to get "on the job exercise"—whether working in the fields or in a factory. Instead, today we must "pay" for our exercise with our leisure time—giving up a piece of our non-working time to exercise—while also contributing a part of our disposable income to gym and health club memberships. Additionally, the cost of calories has also gone down with the rise in agricultural production. In other words, calories are cheaper than ever.

So, it appears, as nations and economies develop, so do waistlines.

Economic Scene; New York Times; Thursday, March 22, 2001

5

moderate activity, such as brisk walking, or gardening each day), we can help decrease obesity and prevent the many serious chronic diseases that are associated with it. The Surgeon General found that "Americans can substantially improve their health and quality of life by including moderate amounts of physical activity in their daily lives."

Some of the major conclusions of the report follow:

- **People of all ages benefit from regular physical activity.**

- **Incorporating just a moderate amount of physical activity (30 minutes of walking, 15 minutes of running) into your day can result in significant health benefits.**

- **Greater amounts of physical activity can lead to even greater health benefits.**

- **Physical activity reduces the risk of premature death, and of coronary heart disease, high-blood pressure, colon cancer, and diabetes. It is good for the muscles, bones and joints, and promotes better mental health as well.**

- **Physical activity declines dramatically during adolescence.**

In essence the report was a wake-up call to get America moving and losing (fat, that is.) Unfortunately, it's five years later and it appears that we are still asleep (and Sleeping Beauties we're not!) Nearly 60 percent of us remain inactive!

In the wake of all this, The CDC calls for a national effort to be launched to fight fat. Says Koplan: *"Obesity is an epidemic and should be taken as seriously as an infectious disease epidemic."*

6

That's a serious statement, not just for the health and fitness of each of us, but for the fitness of our country as well. Did you know that just by becoming more active we could save the nation $76.6 billion dollars in health-care related costs! So by losing fat and increasing your physical activity you will not only be helping yourself, you also will be doing a great service to your country.

More Scientific Evidence

In 1995, The National Heart, Lung, and Blood Institute, in cooperation with the National Institute of Diabetes and Digestive and Kidney Diseases released evidence-based guidelines for health professionals to treat the obesity crisis.

These guidelines include the following:

- **You are at risk for developing obesity-related diseases such as hypertension and high-blood pressure if your body mass index (BMI) is 25 or over (BMI is a relative weight based on height measure of obesity and will be explained later).**

- **Treating obesity should focus on both altering dietary and physical activity patterns.**

- **Obesity is clearly associated with increased sickness and death and losing fat reduces this increased risk.**

- **Experience reveals that lost weight usually will be regained unless the program includes dietary therapy, physical activity and behavior therapy.**

- **Physical activity is integral to a fat loss/weight control program. All adults should set a long-term goal to accumulate at least 30 minutes or more of**

7

physical activity on most, preferably all days of the
week.

- Combining a reduced-calorie diet with physical
activity is recommended to decrease abdominal fat
and increase cardio respiratory fitness.

So...what does all this mean for you?

Well, unfortunately, none of the popular trendy fad diets has been able to
put a lid on public enemy number one: fat. Most diets focus on how much
you weigh, on losing pounds. These diets proudly claim you can lose 10
pounds in two weeks. They may be right. When a diet severely restricts
calories or eliminates certain nutrients (like the ultra-low carbohydrate
diets) you will lose a lot of weight initially. The problem is that most of the
weight lost will be water or lean muscle—not fat. And, since very restrictive diets are nearly impossible to adhere to long-term (not to mention
unhealthy), most people will gain all the weight back; and what they often
gain back is fat. *In fact, the media recently reported that these fad diets
simply don't work.* So the last thing we need is another trendy diet or the
promise of a magic pill that will shrink fat away. What we do need is to
make sense of the solid, scientifically-backed information available, which
is based on the weight management guidelines and physical activity recommendations of the most credible source around: the U.S. Government.

*Remember, it is in our country's best interest that all of us be healthy
and fit for life!*

Enter Combat Fat!

The premise behind Combat Fat! is that it's your body composition, specifically the amount of body fat that you carry that is the most important part
of your fitness to monitor. Not only does being over-fat place you at risk for

8

a number of serious diseases, it also negatively affects your appearance, self-confidence, and energy level. *The conventional focus on weight rather than on body composition is one of the major problems with traditional diets.*

Why? Because your weight is not an accurate indicator of how fat you are. This may sound strange to you now, but we will explain it thoroughly. For now, know that there are "heavy" people who may weigh in with a big number on the scale, but who, in fact, have small percentages of fat on their body. They are fit. Likewise, there are "thin" people who don't weigh much but whose percentage of body fat is unhealthily high.

Combat Fat! is not a diet. It is not a fad. It is a comprehensive holistic approach, based on the government's recommendations, to help you fight fat, and develop a healthy living plan that you can and will want to maintain forever—not just for a few weeks or months. In essence we will help you to effectively change your lifestyle—your mental outlook, habits, food choices—so that you can live a more healthy, fit life.

The premise behind Combat Fat! is that it's the amount of BODY FAT that you carry that is the most important part of your fitness to monitor. It is a comprehensive approach, based on the government's recommendations, to help you develop a healthy living plan that you can and will want to maintain forever!

9

However, it's not so easy to change. Humans are creatures of habit, and most change is often a difficult process. People tend to gravitate toward routines, whether they be the types of foods they eat, or what they do in leisure time. Imagine how challenging it is to actually alter your lifestyle! To help you do this, we look at cognitive, behavioral and physical aspects of behavior change. First we address the cognitive (mental) and behavioral issues around being over-fat. Researchers have found that having a positive attitude and high level of motivation are essential in order for us to succeed at any kind of behavioral change. Of course there also are obstacles, or barriers (such as emotional eating) that can undermine the most committed person. Fortunately, there are many well-regarded strategies to help you successfully overcome these barriers and make important changes in your behavior.

In this book you will learn how you can prepare yourself mentally for change. You will be able to recognize and understand the problems and solutions involved in combating fat. You also will learn how to effectively measure and monitor your body fat using the easy skin-fold caliper method. **The weight-loss focus of Combat Fat! is on FAT just the FAT—not on how much you weigh. You'll find that numbers on the scale can be extremely misleading. In fact we tell you to throw out the scale.** Toss it! Turn it into a plant holder. Just don't get on it again. You'll experience faster, longer lasting results when you focus on your fat instead of on your weight. Combat Fat!, and your weight will follow. Finally, you will learn how to develop a habit of health that includes healthy eating, a positive mental outlook and a more active lifestyle.

> # You'll experience faster, longer lasting results when you focus on your FAT instead of on your WEIGHT.

We want to make this as easy as possible for you, so we provide all the tools you need including a **free skin-fold caliper** to measure and monitor your body fat in a simple one-step procedure, a comprehensive 60-day eating plan with tasty, healthy dishes you and your family will love, and which do away with all the cumbersome calorie and gram counting, and a workout plan tailored to your current level of fitness.

Best of all, you can be assured that the eating and exercising approaches we present are based on valid scientific research into what really works long-term. They are grounded in research and advice from several government agencies and offices including the Department of Health and Human Services, Food and Drug Administration (FDA), Centers for Disease Control and Prevention, and the U.S. Surgeon General. Whether you are a sedentary person with low fitness, or someone who wants to improve your fitness and take it to the next level Combat Fat! has a targeted program designed to help you successfully achieve your fitness goals.

2
Combat Fat!
The Mission

This chapter provides you with an understanding of fat. Yes, in order to defeat the enemy, you must know the enemy. And to know fat is to love fat too. Love fat? Well, not too much but enough to know that your body needs some fat to live long and prosper. Just as too much fat is unhealthy, too little fat is unhealthy too.

For years, body fat measurements have been viewed as esoteric—the realm of high performance athletes and body builders—definitely not for the rest of us.

Well much has changed in recent years, including the development of reliable body fat measuring devices—commonly referred to as skin-fold calipers. We will teach you how to use calipers to self-assess and self-monitor your body fat percentages. Once you've learned to use the calipers and interpret their meaning on the charts, you'll be able to track your progress on a weekly, bi-weekly, or monthly cycle, according to your needs.

We emphasize the skin-fold caliper measurement over the weight measurement for one basic reason: the caliper measurement is a more accurate indicator of your body fat percentage. When you hop on a scale, you are measuring everything; bones, organs, skin, water, muscles, and fat. When you measure fat you measure only that—fat.

WHAT IS BODY FAT?

As we've said before, the Combat Fat! program was designed to address the obesity crisis in America. Its goal is to help you to successfully achieve a healthy, fit body composition by changing lifestyle habits that may have been preventing you from looking and feeling your best. The focus of the weight loss component of our program is on fat loss, rather than pound loss, as in traditional diets. The reason for this shift will be made clear. But first let's differentiate between "fat" the nutrient that we get from our diet; and the body fat that we carry around our waist, hips and thighs.

Fat in Food

As a nutrient, fat has been most misunderstood. For years, especially during the high-carbohydrate craze, it was vilified, to be avoided at all costs, equated to Satan in its capacity for evil. We were told the less fat we eat the better, and were bombarded by a proliferation of low- and non-fat foods, many of which, although low in fat, were highly caloric. Unfortunately, many of us stuffed ourselves with these foods in the mistaken belief that because they contained no fat, we would not *get* fat.

Well, we got fat. We ate too many calories of nonfat foods—and so much of it was in the form of unrefined sugars. These extra calories may have led to the widespread increase in a condition known as Syndrome X—which is characterized by a decreased tolerance for glucose as well as high blood pressure and increased abdominal fat. People with Syndrome X are at higher risk for developing cardiovascular disease and diabetes.

Today, there is a more balanced recognition that we in fact need some fat in our diets—that a combination of a moderate amount fat, along with carbohydrates and protein is optimal for our health. But you need to choose your fats wisely, and in the right quantities. You'll find detailed information on fat and your diet in the Combat Fat! Nutrition section this book.

14

Fat on your Body

Let's shift now from the nutrient fat to the fat that we carry on our bodies. We all have body fat (known technically as adipose tissue). We all must have some body fat. It is not only the body's primary energy reserve (think Tom Hanks in the movie *Castaway*—imagine if he had had absolutely no body fat during those first few weeks on the island!), it also provides insulation from the cold, and protects the organs. Women who have too little body fat risk a condition known as amenorrhea in which their menstrual cycle shuts down, and may be at increased risk for infertility and osteoporosis. The point is that you should not hate body fat. Instead, recognize that it is one of the essential parts of our anatomy, along with the muscles, organs, bones and everything else. It's not a question of whether we should have body fat; rather, it's a matter of how much fat we have. And too many of us have too much!

Body fat is distributed differently on all of us; some of this is due to genetics. (You know how you see your mother's thighs or dad's gut in the mirror!) Where you tend to store fat can directly impact your health. *The worst place to store fat is around the abdominal area; since this is associated with greater risk of coronary artery disease and death.*

Exercise specialists break our bodies down into two distinct parts; fat weight and lean body mass. Lean body mass, also called fat-free mass, is everything other than fat and includes the muscles, organs, bones, blood, connective tissues, etc. So when we talk about your percentage of fat-free mass it simply is the percentage of your body that is not comprised of fat. This is the percentage that most of us need to increase! Likewise, most of us need to decrease our percentage of body fat. Combat Fat! will show you how.

Body Fat vs. Weight

Why focus on body fat rather than weight? After all, if you lose ten pounds

15

that's great isn't it? The answer to that question is a qualified "maybe" because it depends on where those ten pounds came from. When we shed pounds we automatically think that we are losing fat, but it is equally possible that five of the pounds lost were from water. Who wants to lose water? Worse yet, if you are on a very restrictive diet and do not exercise your body can actually lose lean mass—absolutely not what you want to do.

Traditionally, we have judged ourselves to be "fat" or "thin" based on our weight. We've looked at charts that tell us how much we should weigh for our age or height and are aghast if the number falls above the given range.

However, these types of measures have serious shortcomings because they don't take into consideration what comprises that weight. Is it primarily fat or lean mass? This distinction is crucial and is what you will be concerned with on the Combat Fat! program. It's like the difference between a gold-plated necklace and one made of solid gold; they may feel the same, but there are huge distinctions in quality.

For example, you may know some people who, after a few weeks of strength training, report that while their weight has remained the same on the scale, their clothes fit better and they may actually have dropped a size. They have lost fat, while at the same time gained muscle (lean) body mass. The number on the scale hasn't changed but their bodies sure have, and for the better!

The Body Mass Index (BMI)

The government uses what is called the Body Mass Index or BMI to determine obesity. BMI is considered more useful than the standard height/weight tables, such as those on the Metropolitan Life Charts, because it uses a formula to calculate an index based on the ratio of your weight to your height squared. People with normal weight ranges usually have a BMI between 19 and 25 (see chart). Anyone with a BMI greater than 25 is considered overweight and over

16

30 is considered obese. BMI is useful because you can quickly refer to the chart to see where you fall to get a sense of whether you have a weight problem.

The problem with BMI is that it tells you nothing about the composition of your body: how much is fat, how much is muscle. *In fact, the American College of Sports Medicine recommends* **not** *to use BMI to determine your actual "fatness"!*

To really know the composition of your body you need to go a step further and actually measure your body fat. Combat Fat! will show you how to easily and accurately determine your body composition.

All this does not mean that you won't actually lose weight on the Combat Fat! program. Many of you will, especially if you are more than slightly over-fat to begin with. There is a definite association between weight and fat; and you can generally say the more you weigh the fatter you probably are. (After all, very few people who weigh more than 250 pounds can claim that they have healthy percentages of body fat.)

The key concept to take away is that percentage of body fat is a more important and significant indicator of your overall fitness than your weight. And if you successfully lose body fat, you can rest assured that you will look and feel better than ever.

So our advice? Throw out your scales! Instead, learn how to easily and accurately measure your body fat percentage and weight loss from fat will follow. Only by measuring your body fat can you truly know you are changing your body composition for the better.

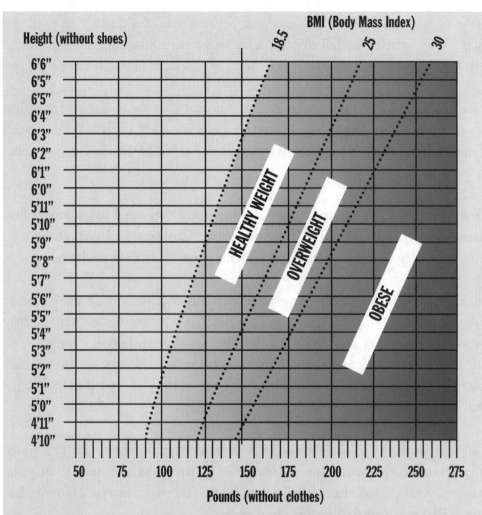

Height (without shoes)

BMI (Body Mass Index)

18.5   25   30

HEALTHY WEIGHT

OVERWEIGHT

OBESE

6'6"
6'5"
6'5"
6'4"
6'3"
6'2"
6'1"
6'0"
5'11"
5'10"
5'9"
5"8"
5'7"
5'6"
5'5"
5'4"
5'3"
5'2"
5'1"
5'0"
4'11"
4'10"

50   75   100   125   150   175   200   225   250   275

Pounds (without clothes)

BMI measures weight in relation to height. The BMI ranges shown above are for adults. They are not exact ranges of healthy and unhealthy weights. However, they show that health risk increases at higher levels of overweight and obesity. Even within the healthy BMI range, weight gains can carry health risks for adults.

Directions: Find your weight on the bottom of the graph. Go straight up from that point until you come to the line that matches your height. Then look to find your weight group.

Healthy Weight: BMI from 18.5 up to 25 refers to a healthy weight.
Overweight: BMI from 25 up to 30 refers to overweight.
Obese: BMI 30 or higher refers to obesity. Obese persons are also overweight.

18

How You Get Body Fat

Body fat is formed whenever we have an energy imbalance in which the energy we take in is greater than the energy that we expend. Energy in the body is measured in calories. A calorie is the energy required to raise one ml of water one degree Celsius. Anytime we do anything, even sitting or sleeping we are expending some energy, just to keep our bodies functioning. You've probably heard the saying, energy in = energy out. This means that if you burn the exact amount of energy you expend in a day you will neither gain nor lose fat. Likewise, if you burn less energy than you take in through food, you will get fat.

How You Lose Body Fat

Conversely, if you take in fewer calories than you burn you will lose fat. In other words, you need to create what is known as a negative calorie balance. The American College of Sports Medicine recommends that in order to lose body fat, you both increase the number of calories burned by doing exercise as well as decrease the number of calories you consume. Exercise is a vital component to this because remember, you want to lose body fat not lean mass. If you were to just scale back on your eating and strictly reduce your caloric intake without exercising, you would actually lose more fat-free tissue and less fat! So while you may have lost "weight" a significant amount of this lost weight may have come from the lean tissue of your body. This is just the opposite of what we want to do in Combat Fat! In Combat Fat! we want to target the fat in your body—just the fat and nothing but the fat!

Studies have shown that you cannot actually decrease the number of fat cells that you carry, but that you can decrease the diameter of those cells through a good nutrition and exercise program. This is why it is so important to make sure that young people have a healthy eating and exercise lifestyle, so that they don't develop fat cells during their youth.

19

According to the American Council on Exercise, the best way to reduce your percentage of body fat is to significantly increase your DAILY CALORIC EXPENDITURE through exercise and to eat a SENSIBLE DIET.

So in order to decrease your total body fat, you need to create a negative energy balance: you need to burn more energy in a day than you take in through food. Since one pound of a fat equals approximately 3500 calories; if you wanted to decrease your fat by one pound a week you would need to create an energy deficit of about 500 calories per day through both a reduction in food intake and an increase in physical activity. Remember, changing your food intake alone truly is not enough!

You'll want to do both cardiovascular exercise and strength training for exercise. Cardiovascular training is good for the health of your heart and lungs, and as a way to burn many calories. Strength training is also a vital component of your exercise program, because it helps to build lean mass. Lean mass burns fat at rest (when you are watching tv for example). So the leaner you are, the more fat you will be burning each and every day, even when you are not exercising.

According to the American Council on Exercise the best way to reduce your percentage of body fat is to significantly increase your daily caloric expenditure through exercise and to eat a sensible diet. Not sexy or earth shattering, but true.

20

.combat-fat.com www.combat-fat.com www.combat-fat.com www.combat-fat.com www.combat-fat.

Weight Adjustment Supplements: Fact Vs. Whacked

"Lose weight while you sleep." "Eat all you want and watch the fat fall off." "This pill will make you look like you've been working out for years." "Flush fat out of the body."

We've all seen the enticing ads. Weight loss and gain supplements, potions, and gadgets are now almost as popular as diet books, but do they work? Time to separate the "fat from the skinny."

The Food and Drug Administration has now banned over 100 ingredients previously found in over-the-counter diet products from the marketplace because they failed to induce weight loss or suppress the appetite.

Although ineffective for weight loss, supplements including **spirulina** (a type of blue-green algae), **lecithin**, **starch blockers**, **fat blockers**, **magnet pills**, **glucommannan**, **skin diet patches**, and **coenzyme Q10** do promote a big, fat cash loss! Let's explore a few other substances in greater detail.

You name it, **kombucha tea** is claimed to cure it. In addition to burning body fat, this product is said to cure AIDS, cancer and so on. Not only is this product ineffective, it might be dangerous. Claims of liver damage, allergic reactions, drug interactions and death have been reported.

Ephedra, also known as ephedrine, pseudoephrine, ma huang and epitonin, is another potentially fatal ingredient in weight-loss supplements. It can raise blood pressure, injure muscles, and induce nerve damage, psychosis, memory loss and stroke. It also has been linked to several deaths.

21

Carnitine is a substance produced by the body. Consuming more via supplements does not improve athletic endurance or improve fat burning ability.

Product marketers suggest **chromium picolinate** builds muscle and helps you lose weight. The truth is that the claims haven't panned out in the research lab. Furthermore, since chromium is indestructible by the body, excess ingestion may have serious health risks.

Amino acids and **protein powders** have been marketed as a cure for obesity, insomnia, pain and depression. More often though, they have been pushed as muscle builders. As stated earlier, an overabundance of protein doesn't magically build muscle. Excess protein, in fact, is converted to body fat. So, not only will you fail to lose weight or gain muscle, you probably will gain fat.

Creatine is one of the most popular amino acid supplements. This one is said to enhance athletic performance but has failed to show its effectiveness outside of the laboratory setting. Gastrointestinal disturbances and muscle cramping have been reported, but how creatine will affect the body's organ systems over time is of greater concern. The expense of using weight adjustment supplements, in terms of your health and money, far outweighs any unlikely beneficial effects.

Before popping a pill or potion in search of an easy dietary fix, think hard. The "magic pill" isn't in the bottle; it's in the kitchen and gym. Eat reasonably, exercise and your goals will be achieved.

Recently, you may have read about people taking more drastic measures, such as liposuction and other types of surgery in order to reduce their body fat. This approach, while effective initially, contains significant risk (as does all surgery) and has a number of shortcomings, the most significant probably being that the surgical change is not permanent. In other words, if you don't change your lifestyle eating and exercising habits, you will get fat again.

How You Measure Body Fat

An accurate assessment of body composition (meaning how much body fat you carry) is recommended for everyone who wants to start a weight-loss or exercise program. Traditionally, people have used height-weight tables to assess their weight. As we've said before, we want you to throw out the scales, because what you weigh does not accurately represent the composition of your body.

There are several methods to estimate body composition. We'll discuss a few, before going in-depth into our preferred method (because of its ease).

Hydrostatic Weighing. For years hydrostatic (underwater weighing) has been considered the gold standard in determining body fat. This technique is based on the following principle by Archimedes: a body immersed in water is buoyed by a counterforce equal to the weight of the water displaced. Fat is less dense in water; so a person who has less body fat will weigh more when immersed in water and will also have a higher body density. Although this is a very accurate way to measure body fat, it sure isn't easy to do and not practical for most of us.

Plethysmography. This methods measures body volume by air displacement, rather than water. Once body density is determined, percent body fat can be calculated.

Bioelectrical Impedance. This method uses electrodes attached to the hand, wrist foot and ankle to determine body fat because fat free tissue is a good conductor of electrical current, while fat is not. BIA analyzers then calculate body composition based on the electrical current readings.

The three methods mentioned above, while providing pretty accurate estimates of body fat are not easily accessible and certainly cannot be done at home. Convenience and accessibility are key factors in determining whether we will stick with something, especially a weight-loss and exercise program. For this reason Combat Fat! recommends the method most often used by professional personal trainers: taking your skinfold measurement using a skinfold caliper.

Skinfold Measurements. The principle behind the skinfold measurement technique is that the amount of subcutaneous fat you hold (that's the fat right under your skin) is proportional to your total body fat. So, by measuring one, you can estimate the other. The method usually involves measuring your subcutaneous fat at various sites in your body with a caliper—a hand-held instrument that calculates the sum of several skinfolds in an equation with other predictors of body fat—to arrive at an estimate of your total body fat percentage.

The American College of Sports Medicine recently tested the accuracy of a variety of skinfold calipers and determined that the small plastic versions are virtually as accurate as the more expensive metal kind, common in gyms. So you don't need to make a financial investment to measure your body fat.

Traditionally, the sites to measure include the abdomen, bicep, chest, tricep and thigh. It is not necessary to measure all of these sites at one time; however most calipers require you to measure at least three sites. You can have a fitness professional measure your body fat, or you can measure it at home with our caliper of choice.

24

.combat-fat.com www.combat-fat.com www.combat-fat.com www.combat-fat.com www.combat-fat.

The Combat Fat! Skin-Fold Caliper

Since most calipers require elaborate calculations and the measurement of several sites, The Combat Fat! program recommends the Accu-Measure Caliper, which you can receive free by sending in the form found at the end of this book in Appendix.

This caliper is particularly easy to use, since it requires you to measure just one convenient site—the abdomen for men and the iliac crest (just inside your hip) for women. There are no calculations to make. In just one simple step you will have an accurate estimate of your body fat in the privacy of your own home, and be ready to set your fat-loss goals. In addition, you will use the skinfold caliper to monitor your progress on the Combat Fat! Program by completing a weekly log of your body fat percentage.

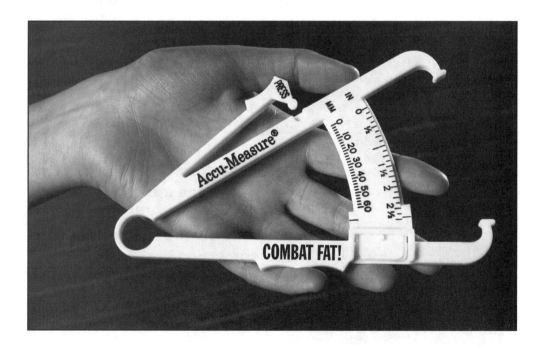

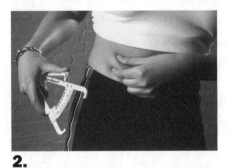
1.

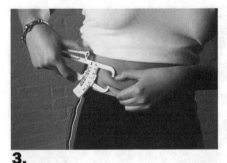
2.

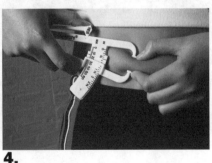
3.

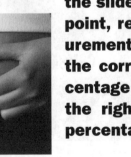
4.

How to Use the Combat Fat! Caliper

You should always take your skinfold measurement before you work out. If you take it right after you exercise, the results will be skewed. Relax as much as possible.

1. Locate the skinfold site on your body.

2. Use your thumb and index finger to grasp the fold and underlying fat. Draw up the fold. Be careful not to pinch so hard that your fingers compress the fat.

3. Make sure the slide on the Accu-Measure Caliper is all the way to the right, then place the caliper over the skinfold.

4. Press. You'll hear a click as the slide goes into place. At that point, read the millimeter measurement on the caliper and find the corresponding body fat percentage on the chart printed to the right. That's your body fat percentage. Simple.

26

BODY FAT INTERPRETATION CHART FOR WOMEN

AGE	SKINFOLD MEASUREMENT IN MILLIMETERS																
	2-3	4-5	6-7	8-9	10-11	12-13	14-15	16-17	18-19	20-21	22-23	24-25	26-27	28-29	30-31	23-33	34-36
UP TO 20	11.3	13.5	15.7	17.7	19.7	21.5	23.2	24.8	26.3	27.7	29.0	30.2	31.3	32.3	33.1	33.9	34.6
21-25	11.9	14.2	16.3	18.4	20.3	22.1	23.8	25.5	27.0	28.4	29.6	30.8	31.9	32.9	33.8	34.5	35.2
26-30	12.5	14.8	16.9	19.0	20.9	22.7	24.5	26.1	27.6	29.0	30.3	31.5	32.5	33.5	34.4	35.2	35.8
31-35	13.2	15.4	17.6	19.6	21.5	23.4	25.1	26.7	28.2	29.6	30.9	32.1	33.2	34.1	35.0	35.8	36.4
36-40	13.8	16.0	18.2	20.2	22.2	24.0	25.7	27.3	28.8	30.2	31.5	32.7	33.8	34.8	35.6	36.4	37.0
41-45	14.4	16.7	18.8	20.8	22.8	24.6	26.3	27.9	29.4	30.8	32.1	33.3	34.4	35.4	36.3	37.0	37.7
46-50	15.0	17.3	19.4	21.5	23.4	25.2	26.9	28.6	30.1	31.5	32.8	34.0	35.0	36.0	36.9	37.6	38.3
51-55	15.6	17.9	20.0	22.1	24.0	25.9	27.6	29.2	30.7	32.1	33.4	34.6	35.6	36.6	37.5	38.3	38.9
56 & UP	16.3	18.5	20.7	22.7	24.6	26.5	28.2	29.8	31.3	32.7	34.0	35.2	36.3	37.2	38.1	38.9	39.5
	LEAN				IDEAL				AVERAGE				OVERFAT				

Data provided by Dr. Andrew S. Jackson (University of Houston) and Dr. Michael L. Pollock (University of Florida).

BODY FAT INTERPRETATION CHART FOR MEN

AGE	SKINFOLD MEASUREMENT IN MILLIMETERS																
	2-3	4-5	6-7	8-9	10-11	12-13	14-15	16-17	18-19	20-21	22-23	24-25	26-27	28-29	30-31	32-33	34-36
UP TO 20	2.0	3.9	6.2	8.5	10.5	12.5	14.3	16.0	17.5	18.9	20.2	21.3	22.3	23.1	23.8	24.3	24.9
21-25	2.5	4.9	7.3	9.5	11.6	13.6	15.4	17.0	18.6	20.0	21.2	22.3	23.3	24.2	24.9	25.4	25.8
26-30	3.5	6.0	8.4	10.6	12.7	14.6	16.4	18.1	19.6	21.0	22.3	23.4	24.4	25.2	25.9	26.5	26.9
31-35	.5	7.1	9.4	11.7	13.7	15.7	17.5	19.2	20.7	22.1	23.4	24.5	25.5	26.3	27.0	27.5	28.0
36-40	5.6	8.1	10.5	12.7	14.8	16.8	18.6	20.2	21.8	23.2	24.4	25.6	26.5	27.4	28.1	28.6	29.0
41-45	6.7	9.2	11.5	13.8	15.9	17.8	19.6	21.3	22.8	24.7	25.5	26.6	27.6	28.4	29.1	29.7	30.1
46-50	7.7	10.2	12.6	14.8	16.9	18.9	20.7	22.4	23.9	25.3	26.6	27.7	28.7	29.5	30.2	30.7	31.2
51-55	8.8	11.3	13.7	15.9	18.0	20.0	21.8	23.4	25.0	26.4	27.6	28.7	29.7	30.6	31.2	31.8	32.2
56 & UP	9.9	12.4	14.7	17.0	19.1	21.0	22.8	24.5	26.0	27.4	28.7	29.8	30.8	31.6	32.3	32.9	33.3
	LEAN				IDEAL				AVERAGE				OVERFAT				

Data provided by Dr. Andrew S. Jackson (University of Houston) and Dr. Michael L. Pollock (University of Florida).

How Much Body Fat Should You Have?

Is your body fat level good or bad? Can it be better? Guidelines for body fat differ for men and women, because women need to have a greater percentage of body fat for reproductive and hormonal reasons. Men have higher natural levels of testosterone which is associated with a greater ability to develop muscles, and therefore, an overall leaner body mass.

In general, to be healthy a woman's body fat percentage should range from 10 percent to 31 percent; body fat percentages for men should range from 2 percent to 25 percent. This rather large range reflects the fact that different percentages of body fat correspond to different levels or classifications of fitness. Keep in mind also that as you age, your body fat percentage most likely will rise, so you need to factor in your age to determine healthy body fat levels.

You can use the following classifications from The American Council on Exercise to help you discover whether you have too much body fat and to determine your body fat percentage goals.

BODY FAT CLASSIFICATION		
CLASSIFICATION	WOMEN (% FAT)	MEN (% FAT)
Essential Fat	10-12%	2-4%
Athletic	14-20	6-13
Fit	21-24	14-17
Acceptable	25-31	18-25
Obese	32+	25+

Source: ACE Lifestyle and Weight Management Consultant Manual (1996) p. 87

28

What if You Have Too Much Body Fat?

After you have used one of the methods described above to determine your percentage of body fat you will be ready to assess your true fitness and determine your goals.

If your body fat levels are too high you need to Combat Fat! *now*. Even if your body fat percentage falls within the acceptable range, you may want to use the Combat Fat! program to increase your fitness. Why not try to go from the acceptable category to fit?

The Combat Fat! Program— It's time to start your mission!

Now that you know all you need to about the importance of using body fat as a measurement of fitness, it's time to commit to Combat Fat! Think of it as a mission you are about to undertake: a "mission: possible" and you're ready to take the first step. You understand the issues involved in changing your diet and physical activity habits, and have the nutrition, exercise and body fat logs ready to help you understand your habits and monitor your progress along the way.

Remember too, that for those times when the program becomes challenging, you have the resources of **www.combat-fat.com** at your disposal. Go there whenever you have a question, or need encouragement to stay on track.

The rewards of successfully completing the Combat Fat! mission are huge: increased health and fitness.

Rest assured that you are not embarking on an untested eccentric diet and weight loss scheme; the program was developed based on the guidelines and recommendations of premier government organizations, including the

Centers for Disease Control, U.S. Surgeon General, and National Institutes of Health.

So it's now up to you. Make a commitment today to the Combat Fat! mission. Measure and record your body fat; determine your goals and then follow the 60-day nutrition and exercise plans in the next two sections of this book, and in the next two months you will be well on your way to a "Mission Accomplished!"

Combat Fat! Quick Start

1. **Measure your body fat percentage with the skin fold caliper and record this baseline percentage in your body fat log.**

2. **Compare your measurement to the Classification Chart above. Bear in mind that the higher end of any range reflects the natural increase in body fat expected with aging. (If, for example, you are 20 years old you can use the lower end of each range as a guideline; if you are 40 you might look mid-range.)**

3. **Determine your body fat goals either on your own or with the assistance of a trainer or registered dietician. Remember to keep the goals realistic and attainable. As a guideline consider that the government recommends a loss of 10 pounds over six months as reasonable.**

4. **Begin the Nutrition and Exercise Components of the Combat Fat! Program. Be sure to monitor and record your dietary and exercise habits daily.**

3
Combat Fat!
Nutrition

When we decided upon the nutritional component of Combat Fat! we had one thing in mind—credibility. It seems that every month brings about a new approach to eating—high carb, low carb, no carb, all fat, fat-free, liquid, solid, animal, vegetable, soy—you name it. Combat Fat! is not about a trendy new diet scheme that will be here today and gone tomorrow. We want our program to work for you today, tomorrow, and in years to come!

We turned to the Dietary Guidelines for Americans *released in 2000 by the U.S. Department of Agriculture and the U.S. Department of Health and Human Services. Why? Because millions of your tax dollars were spent on researching and reviewing the recommendations. Top dietitians and scientists have studied the practicality and reliability of the data. It is tested, supported, credentialed. It works.*

In this chapter you'll learn all about basic nutrition—it's a lesson we can all benefit from. Your daily nutrient needs. Your daily caloric needs. Vitamins, minerals, and more. From there you'll discover the Food Pyramid. It's a simple yet profound way to understand where your calories should come from.

Finally, you'll learn once and for all how to read a nutrition label and be able to make intelligent, healthy decisions at the supermarket or even at a fast food franchise.

The Challenge of Choice

Good nutrition basically boils down to two things: choice and portion. Choice involves the types of foods you eat as well as how those foods are prepared. Are you more apt to eat a baked sweet potato or plate of fries? An apple or apple pie? Even the simplest of choices, such as forgoing slabs of butter on your pancakes, can save you hundreds of calories that you probably won't even miss taste-wise. In the Combat Fat! Plan you learn how to choose healthy, vitamin-packed options, prepared in ways that skimp on calories but not on taste.

> **Eating a variety of foods ensures that you will get all the IMPORTANT NUTRIENTS, VITAMINS, AND MINERALS that is required for optimal health.**

Equally important is how much of each food you eat. There really is no good or bad food (with the exception of trans fatty acids, which we cover later). The key is in portion control. In the last few years portion sizes of virtually all foods—from mega-muffins, to "big grab" chips to cookies to restaurant entrees—have ballooned. Often, what is sold in single packages really represent two or three servings! Combat Fat! shows you how to determine sensible portion sizes based on the Pyramid model. Much of the principles of the Combat Fat! Nutrition Plan are based on the *Dietary Guidelines for Americans* released in 2000 by the U.S. Department of Agriculture and the U.S. Department of Health and Human Services.

This proven nutritional plan includes three major themes: aiming for fitness, building a healthy base and choosing sensibly. It gives you the freedom to choose from many healthful and great tasting foods.

32

There are ten main guidelines in the Dietary Guidelines for Americans:

1. Aim for a healthy weight.

2. Be physically active each day.

3. Let the Pyramid guide your food choices.

4. Choose a variety of grains, in particular whole grains.

5. Choose a variety of fruits an vegetables.

6. Keep food safe.

7. Choose a diet low in saturate fat and cholesterol and moderate in total fat.

8. Choose beverages and foods that are not high in sugar.

9. Choose and prepare foods with less salt.

10. Drink alcoholic beverages only in moderation.

Common Dieting Myths

Many fad diets promote quick weight loss but the loss is not primarily fat. It is chiefly a loss in water and muscle so that pounds return once a sensible diet is resumed. Identifying unsound claims is not easy. However, if it sounds too good to be true, it probably is! If the plan includes one or more of the following claims, be wary.

A quick weight loss of five or more pounds weekly. To lose five pounds in a week you would essentially need to fast. Furthermore, the loss would be primarily water, and weight loss would slow after the first week.

Limited food choices. Not only do these plans fail to meet your nutrient needs, they also foster boredom and the diet quickly gets discarded.

Claims that one food will destroy the calories in another. This claim is ridiculous; a calorie is a calorie!

Promises little or no effort involved. If this were true, no one would have a weight problem.

Boasts that it has been suppressed by the medical profession. There are few conspiracies in science. If you discovered the "fountain of thinness," don't you think the world would be talking about it?

Requires you purchase special pills such as vitamin or mineral supplements. In some cases, supplements are wise to ensure adequate nutrient intake. Most people, however, can get what they need following a healthy weight-loss plan.

Statements that the diet is revolutionary. If this were true, you would hear of its potential from scientific researchers while it was being tested.

Nutrition 101

Fad diets come and go, but basic science-backed nutrition advice has remained remarkably consistent. In fact, many reported studies have proven that the best way to lose fat and keep fat off is to follow a plan that is rooted not in a new trend, but in the Department of Agriculture's Food Guide Pyramid. While most of us are excited by new trends and fads, the truth is that they do not work in the long term. What does work is a balanced eating and exercising plan that is based on reasonable and attainable goals.

The key to the Food Guide Pyramid is that it provides a wide range of choices so you can eat a variety of tasty foods. Eating a variety of foods ensures that you will get all the important nutrients, vitamins, and minerals that your body requires for optimal health. It also means that you won't be bored to death because you can select different foods every day. Sure beats eating 20 grapefruits a week!

Before getting into the pyramid itself, let's talk a bit about the nutrients our bodies need. Nutrients are the fuels that drive our bodies, and allow us to develop structurally. **The six major classes of nutrients are protein, carbohydrate, fat, vitamins minerals and water.** Your body requires different amounts of each nutrient in order to function optimally. The following recommended daily amounts are for normal, healthy adults of average size.

Your Daily Nutrient Needs

Proteins: 50-70 grams per day (which should equal 12 to 20 percent of your daily caloric intake).

Carbohydrates: 350-400 gram per day (approximately 55 to 65 percent of your daily intake). If you exercise more than one hour every day you should consume 65 percent of calories from carbs.

35

Fats: 30 to 65 grams per day approximately (approximately 25 to 30 percent of your caloric intake.)

Vitamins and Minerals: as listed in the *Recommended Dietary Allowances* established by the Food and Nutrition Board of the National Academy of Science.

Water: two to three *quarts* a day.

Your Daily Caloric Needs

How many calories do you need to consume each day to maintain or lose weight? In general, to maintain a healthy weight inactive women and older adults require about 1600 calories a day; older children, active women and most men require about 2200 calories and active men about 2800 calories. Many of us are consuming way above our caloric needs.

If you want to lose fat you need to reduce the number of calories that you consume each day. One pound of fat weighs in at 3500 calories. So, in order to lose one pound of fat in a week, you need to shave approximately 500 calories off your daily food intake.

You should note that the above guidelines are averages, based on healthy Americans and represent generalizations. We all have unique characteristics, for example a super slow resting metabolism, that may call for some modification of these guidelines. If you have a health condition, such as diabetes or heart disease, your optimal balance of nutrients can vary. For example a person with diabetes would want to limit his or her carbohydrates and someone with heart disease would further reduce fat intake. If you have a health condition, be sure to go over your nutritional plan with your primary care physician and/or registered dietitian. You can find a registered dietitian on the website for the American Dietetic Association (www.eatright.org).

36

Let the Pyramid Be Your Guide

The food guide pyramid (shown below) provides a visual depiction of the types and quantities of foods you should eat every day. It is broken into six food groups: grains, vegetables, fruits, dairy, proteins, fats and sweets. Most of your diet should come from the foods at the base or bottom of the pyramid (the grains group) and less should come from those at the top (fats, oils and sweets). You'll notice that you can have six to 11 servings of grains each day, which are rich in carbohydrates.

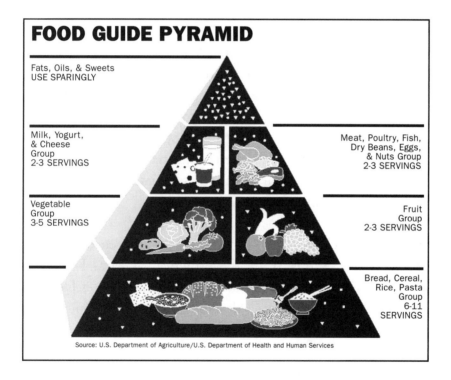

FOOD GUIDE PYRAMID

Fats, Oils, & Sweets
USE SPARINGLY

Milk, Yogurt,
& Cheese
Group
2-3 SERVINGS

Meat, Poultry, Fish,
Dry Beans, Eggs,
& Nuts Group
2-3 SERVINGS

Vegetable
Group
3-5 SERVINGS

Fruit
Group
2-3 SERVINGS

Bread, Cereal,
Rice, Pasta
Group
6-11
SERVINGS

Source: U.S. Department of Agriculture/U.S. Department of Health and Human Services

Popular Diets Analyzed

Not a magazine can be opened nor a bookstore browsed without your eyes being drawn to yet another recommended diet. Current diet book sales are estimated to exceed 140 million dollars yearly. Let's take a look at some of today's most popular regimens.

LOW-CARBOHYDRATE, HIGH-PROTEIN

Just about everyone knows someone who has followed one of the numerous low-carbohydrate, high-protein plans currently being promoted. Initially they seem to work. Weight loss is quick the first week or two, but the loss is primarily water. When your body has exhausted its carbohydrate supply, it manufactures sugar from protein, including muscle protein. Your muscle tissue burns calories like crazy; fat is hardly burned at all. Because of the large amount of muscle loss, caloric needs decrease significantly; weight loss stops, and frustration sets in. When a normal diet is resumed, the pounds return. In many instances, you end up heavier than when the diet was initiated because your metabolic rate decreases along with your muscle loss.

Many low-carbohydrate, high-protein diet books encourage you to ignore recommendations from the American Heart, Dietetic, and Diabetes Associations as well as those of the United States Department of Agriculture. These authorities develop guidelines for optimal health based on extensive scientific research.

Following low-carbohydrate, high-protein plans over the short term can result in constipation, dizziness, irritability, bad breath, improper kidney functioning, a loss of sodium and dehydration. Long-term effects may increase the risk for developing heart attacks, strokes and cancer.

FORMULA DIETS

Various formula diets have been around for years. Most of these do provide adequate nutrition with the exception of dietary fiber. Boredom, however, often sets in quickly and the formula loses its appeal. Since reasonable eating habits were not learned while consuming these low-calorie drinks, the weight is rapidly regained when the formula is abandoned.

HIGH-FIBER DIETS

Many theories lurk behind high-fiber diets. Fiber, when combined with water, causes bulk in the intestines and creates a feeling of fullness. Because most foods rich in fiber take a long time to chew, time available to eat a large quantity of food may be decreased. As a result, fewer calories are consumed. Generally, high fiber foods, such as fruits and vegetables, are low in calories and high in nutrition. Thus, most high-fiber diets are nutritionally sound. Just be sure you also eat adequate amounts of other foods. Let the food pyramid be your guide. Words of caution—don't increase your fiber too rapidly or constipation will set in, and make sure your water consumption rises simultaneously for the same reason.

WEIGHT WATCHERS

The Weight Watchers point and exchange systems promote the intake of a variety of foods and are well balanced. Meal plans are individualized; weight-loss is slow, and behavior modification is taught. Many people also find the group support helpful. The cons include cost and time spent going to weekly meetings.

The Importance of Fruits and Vegetables

In addition to choosing healthy grains, try to eat at least five servings of fruits and vegetables every day. This is essential. Many scientific studies have shown that people who eat diets plentiful in fruits and vegetables have reduced risk for many diseases, including a variety of cancers. Fruits and vegetables are great sources of essential vitamins, minerals and fiber. Unfortunately, most of us do not eat the five recommended servings daily; and if we do, we eat the less healthy vegetables, such as iceberg lettuce, rather than the nutrient-dense dark greens. Dark green leafy vegetables, deeply colored fruits and beans and peas are very rich in vitamins and minerals. A good rule of thumb is to make your plate as colorful as possible with a variety of vegetables to be sure you are getting all the nutrients you need.

How can you make sure you eat enough from this food group? Choose chopped vegetables as a snack when you feel hungry; or grab an apple instead of a candy bar. Drink juice instead of soda. Make salads with tomatoes, cucumbers, peppers and other vegetables. Soon you'll see how easy it really is to eat those five servings.

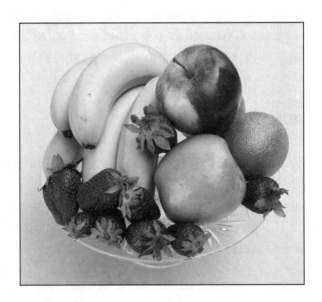

40

Water

Water comprises about 75 percent of our total body weight and it serves many functions. Water helps regulate our body temperature. When we sweat, we rid ourselves of excess heat. Water serves as a transport medium, carrying needed nutrients to our cells and removing toxic substances and wastes. It cushions our body tissues and lubricates our joints. Water provides moisture for our respiratory system and is essential for our digestion. Since water is a major component of all cell structures, including muscle structure and function, it takes second place only to oxygen as the most important body component. Unfortunately, most people often overlook this fact.

Not drinking enough water during exercise or on hot days can result in lack of coordination, irritability, fatigue, muscle cramping, mental confusion and more. Beverages containing alcohol, coffee, tea and many colas are diuretics. They cause our kidneys to excrete more fluid than we normally would. Thus, plain water is the ideal hydration source.

Since we cannot store or conserve water, it is important to make sure that we drink adequate amounts of it every day, especially when it is hot or when we are exercising. In general, you should consume two to three quarts a day (that's eight to twelve 8-ounce glasses). Ideally you should drink water in intervals throughout the day. Try bringing a large bottle to work with you. Keep it at your desk so that you can easily take regular drinks. When you exercise you should drink one to two cups of water an hour before you begin and then an additional four to eight ounces every 15 minutes during your workout. Do not wait until you are thirsty to drink; by then you probably already are in a state of dehydration.

Vitamins & Minerals

When it comes to supplementing our diets with vitamins people get very passionate. Some people have strong beliefs that taking a large number of vitamins each day is necessary to maintain or improve their health. However, vitamins are not subject to the approval of the Food and Drug Administration and manufacturers have wide leeway in marketing these products. You should be careful about taking any vitamins in very large doses (100 times the RDA) as they can be toxic at these levels.

Vitamins and minerals are found in the foods that we eat and most nutrition experts agree that the best way to get vitamins is through a healthy diet. After all, our bodies were meant to absorb vitamins through food, not in pill form. So, if you eat a healthy diet based on the pyramid guidelines you probably will get all the vitamins and minerals you need. However, many of us because of poor eating habits, have developed deficiencies—most often in folate, vitamin B6 , antioxidants, calcium and zinc. Taking a simple multivitamin once a day that does not exceed the recommended nutrient levels is a good way to insure that you are receiving adequate amounts of these nutrients.

Make sure you get enough antioxidants because these compounds preserve and protect your body's cells from the damage of free radicals. Free radicals are oxygen molecules that have split into single electron molecules, which can cause health problems because of the damage they do to tissues. Beta carotene, vitamins C and E, and the minerals sulfur and selenium are strong antioxidants. The following chart provides the US RDA for the major vitamins and minerals for adults and children over four. Bear in mind that your age and certain health conditions (including pregnancy) may call for you to have more or less of a particular vitamin or mineral. Check with your doctor.

VITAMIN A

FUNCTIONS	prevents night blindness, keeps body tissues healthy, allows for normal bone and teeth growth
BEST FOOD SOURCES	dark green leafy vegetables, red, orange or yellow vegetables and fruits, liver, eggs, fish oils, and fortified foods such as milk
REQUIREMENTS	800 to 1000 microgram retinol equivalents
DEFICIENCY	poor night vision, increased risk of osteomalacia (soft bones), and osteoporosis
TOXICITY	liver damage, bone abnormalities, headaches, double vision, hair loss, vomiting

VITAMIN D

FUNCTIONS	promotes strong bones and teeth
BEST FOOD SOURCES	eggs, cheese, sardines, fortified milk, cereals and margarine
REQUIREMENTS	5 to 10 micrograms
DEFICIENCY	increased osteoporosis and osteomalacia risk
TOXICITY	Weak muscles and bones, kidney stones and damage, excessive bleeding

VITAMIN E

FUNCTIONS	helps form cell membranes, increases resistance to disease and possibly reduces the risk of certain cancers as well as heart disease
BEST FOOD SOURCES	vegetable oils, seeds, nuts and wheat germ
REQUIREMENTS	8 to 10 mg alpha-tocopherol equivalents
DEFICIENCY	abnormal nervous system functioning, premature very-low birthweight infants
TOXICITY	unknown but very high amounts may interfere with the functioning of other nutrients

VITAMIN K

FUNCTIONS	promotes normal blood clotting
BEST FOOD SOURCES	green leafy vegetables
REQUIREMENTS	55 to 80 micrograms
DEFICIENCY	abnormal blood clotting
TOXICITY	none known

43

VITAMIN C

FUNCTIONS	repairs damaged tissues, promotes wound healing, increases resistance to infection, maintains healthy gums, bones, and teeth
BEST FOOD SOURCES	citrus fruits and juices, strawberries, tomatoes, potatoes and raw cabbage
REQUIREMENTS	60 milligrams
DEFICIENCY	scurvy (symptoms may include bleeding, improper wound healing, loose teeth, and swollen gums)
TOXICITY	gastrointestinal pain and diarrhea

VITAMIN B1 (THIAMIN)

FUNCTIONS	carbohydrate metabolism
BEST FOOD SOURCES	whole grains, nuts, peas, beans, pork, enriched breads and cereals
REQUIREMENTS	1 to 1.5 micrograms
DEFICIENCY	weak muscles, nerve damage, fatigue
TOXICITY	none known

VITAMIN B2 (RIBOFLAVIN)

FUNCTIONS	energy release and cell repair
BEST FOOD SOURCES	poultry, enriched breads, cereals and grains, as well as green leafy vegetables, organ meats, cheese, milk, and eggs
REQUIREMENTS	1.2 to 1.8 milligrams
DEFICIENCY	sore red tongue, dry flaky skin, cataracts
TOXICITY	none known

NIACIN (NICOTINIC ACID)

FUNCTIONS	allows cells to use fuel and oxygen
BEST FOOD SOURCES	meat, fish, poultry, nuts, legumes, enriched cereals and whole grains
REQUIREMENTS	13 to 20 milligrams
DEFICIENCY	pellagra (symptoms may include dermatitis, diarrhea, and dementia)
TOXICITY	in very high doses, flushed skin, possible liver damage, high blood sugar and stomach ulcers

VITAMIN B6 (PYRIDOXINE)

FUNCTIONS assists in protein and red blood cell formation, helps produce antibodies and hormones.

BEST FOOD SOURCES meat, chicken, fish, organ meats, nuts, legumes, and whole grains

REQUIREMENTS 1.5 to 2 milligrams

DEFICIENCY dermatitis, anemia, convulsions, and nausea

TOXICITY nerve damage

FOLATE (FOLACIN OR FOLIC ACID)

FUNCTIONS produces DNA and RNA to make cells, helps make red blood cells

BEST FOOD SOURCES dark green leafy vegetables, orange juice, dried beans, liver, whole grain breads and cereals

REQUIREMENTS 180 to 200 micrograms

DEFICIENCY increased risk of spina bifida in offspring, weakness, irritability, sore red tongue, diarrhea, weight loss, anemia

TOXICITY can mask B12 deficiency, which if untreated, can cause permanent nerve damage

VITAMIN B12 (COBALAMIN)

FUNCTIONS assists in DNA, RNA and nerve formation, helps make red blood cells, facilitates energy metabolism

BEST FOOD SOURCES meat, poultry, fish, dairy products and fortified foods

REQUIREMENTS 2 micrograms

DEFICIENCY numb hands and feet, fatigue, anemia

TOXICITY none known

BIOTIN

FUNCTIONS assists in energy production

BEST FOOD SOURCES eggs, liver, dried beans, nuts, whole grains and cereals

REQUIREMENTS 30 to 100 micrograms

DEFICIENCY loss of appetite, fatigue, dry skin, heart abnormalities and depression

TOXICITY none known

PANTOTHENIC ACID

FUNCTIONS	assists in energy production
BEST FOOD SOURCES	meat, poultry, fish, whole grains and legumes
REQUIREMENTS	4 to 7 milligrams
DEFICIENCY	numb hands and feet
TOXICITY	diarrhea and water retention

Minerals

CALCIUM

FUNCTIONS	required for blood clotting, nerve, muscle and cell membrane functions, builds bone and teeth, promotes enzyme reactions
BEST FOOD SOURCES	dairy products, green leafy vegetables, tofu, almonds and legumes
REQUIREMENTS	800 to 1200 milligrams
DEFICIENCY	increases risk for osteoporosis
TOXICITY	kidney stones and damage, constipation

PHOSPHORUS

FUNCTIONS	promotes bone, teeth, DNA and RNA growth, assists in energy production
BEST FOOD SOURCES	meat, poultry, fish, eggs, legumes, nuts and breads
REQUIREMENTS	800 to 1200 milligrams
DEFICIENCY	bone loss, weakness, loss of appetite and pain
TOXICITY	decreases calcium levels in the blood leading to bone loss

MAGNESIUM

FUNCTIONS	component of bones and many enzymes, needed for energy production, muscle contractions, normal nerve and muscle cell functioning
BEST FOOD SOURCES	whole grains, legumes, nuts
REQUIREMENTS	280 to 400 milligrams
DEFICIENCY	muscle tremors, poor coordination, nausea, weakness, convulsions and poor appetite
TOXICITY	nausea, low blood pressure, heart abnormalities, vomiting

CHROMIUM

FUNCTIONS	allows body to use glucose
BEST FOOD SOURCE	nuts, whole grains and meat
REQUIREMENTS	50 to 200 micrograms
DEFICIENCY	nerve damage and high blood sugar
TOXICITY	none known

COPPER

FUNCTIONS	facilitates energy production, component of enzymes, helps form hemoglobin and connective tissue
BEST FOOD SOURCES	fruits, vegetables, nuts, seeds, legumes, liver
REQUIREMENTS	1.5 to 3 milligrams
DEFICIENCY	anemia
TOXICITY	liver damage, coma, nausea, vomiting and diarrhea

FLOURIDE

FUNCTIONS	prevents tooth decay, strengthens bones
BEST FOOD SOURCES	sardines, salmon, fluoridated water and tea
REQUIREMENTS	1.5 to 4 milligrams
DEFICIENCY	tooth decay
TOXICITY	brittle bones, stained or mottled teeth

IODINE

FUNCTIONS	forms hormones that regulate the rate of energy usage
BEST FOOD SOURCES	seafood and table salt
REQUIREMENTS	150 micrograms
DEFICIENCY	enlarged thyroid and weight gain
TOXICITY	enlarged thyroid

IRON

FUNCTIONS	component of hemoglobin that carries oxygen to the cells
BEST FOOD SOURCES	meat, poultry, fish, legumes, green leafy vegetables, dried fruits and legumes
REQUIREMENTS	10 to 15 milligrams
DEFICIENCY	infections, anemia and fatigue
TOXICITY	poisons children; may lead to hemochromatosis

47

MANGANESE

FUNCTIONS	a component of enzymes involved in energy and protein metabolism
BEST FOOD SOURCES	whole grain products, tea, fruits and vegetables
REQUIREMENTS	2 to 5 milligrams
DEFICIENCY	rare
TOXICITY	nerve damage

MOLYBDENUM

FUNCTIONS	component of enzymes
BEST FOOD SOURCES	organ meats, milk, legumes and whole grains
REQUIREMENTS	75 to 250 micrograms
DEFICIENCY	rare
TOXICITY	may interfere with copper use

SELENIUM

FUNCTIONS	protects cells from damage, assists with cell growth
BEST FOOD SOURCES	seafood, meats, grains and seeds
REQUIREMENTS	50 to 70 micrograms
DEFICIENCY	may damage the heart
TOXICITY	nerve damage, fatigue, irritability, nausea, vomiting, diarrhea, stomach pain

ZINC

FUNCTIONS	needed for wound healing, growth, reproduction, carbohydrate, protein and alcohol metabolism, and the making of DNA and RNA
BEST FOOD SOURCES	meat, liver, eggs, dairy, whole grains, legumes and oysters
REQUIREMENTS	12 to 15 milligrams
DEFICIENCY	loss of taste, smell and appetite, reduced resistance to infection, scaly skin, growth retardation
TOXICITY	interferes with copper absorption and immune functioning, reduces good blood cholesterol (HDL), upsets stomach and may cause nausea and vomiting

SODIUM

FUNCTIONS	regulates fluids, blood pressure, nerve and muscle function
BEST FOOD SOURCES	processed foods and table salt
REQUIREMENTS	a minimum of 500 milligrams
DEFICIENCY	muscle cramps, dizziness, nausea and fatigue
TOXICITY	may cause high blood pressure

POTASSIUM

FUNCTIONS	fluid and mineral balance, blood pressure regulation, nerve and muscle function
BEST FOOD SOURCES	fruits, vegetables, poultry, meat and fish
REQUIREMENTS	a minimum of 2000 milligrams
DEFICIENCY	abnormal heartbeat, muscle paralysis, weakness, lethargy
TOXICITY	heart abnormalities

CHLORIDE

FUNCTIONS	component of stomach acid, regulates fluid balance
BEST FOOD SOURCES	table salt
REQUIREMENTS	a minimum of 750 milligrams
DEFICIENCY	growth failure, behavioral and learning problems, poor appetite
TOXICITY	may cause high blood pressure

The Fat-Free Myth

You'll notice that the pyramid guide allows you to consume 25 to 30 percent of your daily calories from fat. What's going on here? For too long we bought into the myth that fat is evil and as long as we severely cut our fat intake, we would also control our waistlines. This was based largely on the fact that high-fat foods contain more calories per gram than do other foods. (A single gram of fat has 9 calories; compared to only 4 calories per gram of carbohydrate and protein). However, substituting non-fat or low-fat products for fats has not led to success in fat loss. Why? Here are the facts about fat:

FACT: Fat-free does not equal calorie-free. Many no-fat or low-fat foods have very high levels of sugar, which can up the calorie content of foods significantly. In addition, there is a tendency for people to eat larger portions of fat-free foods, thereby increasing the amount of calories consumed.

FACT: Fat satiates. In general, you need to eat less of a food with fat than you do of a non-fat food in order to feel full. For this reason, many people tend to overeat non-fat or low-fat foods.

FACT: You NEED some Fat. This one is hard for people to really accept. But it is true. Fat is a major nutrient that is vital for proper growth and development and to maintain good health. Certain vitamins (A,C,E, and K) are soluble only in fat. The Combat Fat! Nutrition Plan, which is based on the Food Pyramid, recommends that approximately 25-30 percent of your daily diet come from fats.

However, not all fats are created equal. In general, you want to steer clear of saturated fats, such as butter and the fat found in meats, along with palm and coconut oils. This is the artery-clogging fat. You should also avoid trans-fatty acids (fats that are formed when foods are hydrogenated, and are found in deep fried commercial foods and many packaged foods, especially baked goods). These fats act like saturated fats—only are they're even worse! In addition to raising levels of bad cholesterol (known as LDL) in our bodies like saturated fats do, they lower the levels of the good cholesterol (HDL) that we need to keep our arteries clear.

The good fats, which are the monosaturated and polyunsaturated kind, (such as olive oil and canola oil) are absolutely necessary for many functions of life. In addition, our bodies require essential fatty acids (EFAs), such as linoleic and alpha linoleic acid, for normal cell growth and development. The only way to get these fatty acids is through your diet. EFAs are found primarily in fatty fish, such as salmon and mackerel, and in certain nuts, oils and dark green vegetables. There is significant evidence that a diet rich in essential fatty acids can protect against heart disease. Recently, the American Heart Association, in recognition of the important heart protective role that these fatty acids play, revised their dietary guidelines to include suggesting that we eat two servings of fatty fish each week.

Reading Food Labels

Have nutritional labels on foods left you confused? Learning how to properly interpret the information presented on a food label gives you a valuable nutrition tool. First, look at the front panel of a food, which lists any foods that have been added. For example, a cereal that has the words "fortified" or "enriched" on the front panel may mean that certain vitamins and/or minerals have been added to the grain. Furthermore, the ingredients listed first are the ones present in the highest concentrations by weight. Too often those ingredients are sugar and sodium. Try to buy foods that have healthy ingredients front and center.

The serving sizes listed on labels can also be misleading. A small bag of potato chips may list "150 calories per serving" and you think "that's not so bad," but you need to carefully read how many servings the bag contains, which often can be two or three. So, if you eat all the chips in a bag that contains three servings, you've actually consumed 450 calories. Not so good.

Finally, it is helpful to know how to convert the nutrients presented on the label in grams to calories in order to determine how much (energy-wise) of each individual nutrient you would be eating in a serving.

Carbohydrates:	**1 gram equals 4 calories**
Proteins:	**1 gram equals 4 calories**
Fats:	**1 gram equals 9 calories.**

When reading labels pay particular attention to the amount of cholesterol and sodium listed. You might be surprised at how many low fat and low calorie foods contain very high levels of sodium (healthy adults should aim for a total intake of no more than 2400 mg per day.) When reading the ingredient list check to see if the food contains any saturated or hydrogenated oils; if it does, you may want to avoid this food since hydrogenated foods contain the unhealthy and potentially harmful trans-fatty acids.

52

Things to Consider
When Reading a Food Label

- Note the order of ingredients listed (those most abundant appear first).

- Read the nutrient information to determine the relative amounts of protein, carbs, fats, vitamins and minerals the food is providing.

- Check the serving size: Beware! Many packages contain two or three servings.

- Avoid foods that contain hydrogenated oils.

- Look for foods that strike a pyramid-based balance among carbohydrates, fats and proteins.

Macaroni & Cheese

Nutrition Facts

Serving Size 1 cup (228g)
Servings Per Container 2

Amount Per Serving

Calories 250 Calories from Fat 110

	% Daily Value*
Total Fat 12g	**18**%
Saturated Fat 3g	**15**%
Cholesterol 30mg	**10**%
Sodium 470mg	**20**%
Total Carbohydrate 31g	**10**%
Dietary Fiber 0g	**0**%
Sugars 5g	
Protein 5g	
Vitamin A	4%
Vitamin C	2%
Calcium	20%
Iron	4%

* Percent Daily Values are based on a 2,000 calorie diet. Your Daily Values may be higher or lower depending on your calorie needs:

	Calories:	2,000	2,500
Total Fat	Less than	65g	80g
Sat Fat	Less than	20g	25g
Cholesterol	Less than	300mg	300mg
Sodium	Less than	2,400mg	2,400mg
Total Carbohydrate		300g	375g
Dietary Fiber		25g	30g

How to Eat Within the System

For most of us it is fairly easy to adhere to a new eating plan when we are preparing our own meals at home. The real challenges come when we eat out (especially at a fast food place.)

Of course you can always bring your lunch from home to ensure that you are eating the most healthfully during your workday. You also should bring bags of cut vegetables such as carrots, or dried fruit, such as small boxes of raisins, for between-meal snacking.

At Your Favorite Restaurant

When at a restaurant, bear in mind the following tips for healthy eating:

- **Choose salads and vegetables from a salad bar or menu (but skip the oily or fat-based dressings).**

- **Ask your waiter how foods are prepared. Are they sautéed, broiled, deep-fried? Stick to those that are broiled, boiled, baked, blackened or stir-fried.**

- **Don't be afraid to ask for your food to be prepared in a lighter, healthier way. Restaurants want your business, and more often than not, are happy to accommodate your needs.**

- **If entrees are large (remember that a portion of meat should be about the size of your palm), consider sharing one with someone. Otherwise, when your food arrives, push half of it off to the side and only eat the other half.**

- **Order fresh fruit or sherbet for dessert.**

- **Watch your consumption of wine; limit yourself to one glass with dinner. And have your drink with**

54

your meal, not beforehand. Alcohol is an appetite stimulant.

Fast Food Franchises

Don't panic if you find yourself at a fast food place. Opt for these more healthy choices:

- **Baked potato (plain) with broccoli.**
- **Lean burger, with no cheese, fries or mayo.**
- **Chicken breast sandwich, without the mayo.**

On the Run Alternatives

Other healthy fast food choices you can quickly eat when you are on the go:

- **Yogurt with fruit**
- **Apple**
- **Handful of nuts**
- **Cut carrots**
- **Raisins**

The 8-Week Combat Fat! Nutrition Plan

While you now know the basics for good nutrition, figuring out how much to eat of what each day may seem daunting. With your day as busy as it is you don't want to have to measure and count calories. That's why we're here. The Combat Fat! Program provides you with an easy to follow 8-week nutrition plan that you can use as a guide in developing your meals. We also have included easy to follow recipes for all of the meals presented in the plan. By following the plan for two months, you will obtain a good sense of the proper portion sizes and food mixes that make up a healthy, nutritious diet. We've figured out all the math for you; you don't have to calcu-

55

late a thing. Best of all, at the end of the 8 weeks, you will be able to eye-ball a meal and determine its nutritional value. Imagine being able to go to a restaurant or friend's home for dinner confident that you will make healthy eating choices! Of course, if you want to continue to follow the eating plan we have laid out for you beyond the 8 weeks, that's fine too. Many of us like to have that kind of specific guidance!

4
Combat Fat! in the Kitchen

When it comes to translating the Food Pyramid, caloric needs, and nutrient needs into a practical plan of eating, there is no one better to do it than a registered dietitian. Your dietitian for the Combat Fat! is M. Laurel "Laurie" Cutlip, LN, RD.

Laurie has devised a brilliantly simple way for you to reduce your caloric and fat intake without sacrificing taste and variety. If it were up to me, I'd suggest that you eat the same way every day. Kind of boring but it keeps the shopping and the cooking predictable.

Laurie presents a portion control system that is easy to follow. Choose a breakfast, choose a lunch, choose a dinner. Add your snacks. Recipes are included too! Fill your cabinets with healthy yummy things. Learn to love spices. Enjoy the cooking process. Make healthy meals for yourself, your friends, and your family.

Indeed I have been known to find something I like and eat it every day. Like grilled chicken breasts. Or steamed spinach with lemon. I once o.d.'d on couscous. But that's another story.

Follow Laurie through the Combat Fat! Kitchen and start cooking healthy today!

Whether you're trying to lose weight, gain weight or simply improve your eating habits, the Combat Fat! nutrition plan will help you reach your goals. What's so special about Combat Fat!? Nothing and everything. There's nothing trendy. No earth shattering "scientific breakthroughs" to report. Just plain old sound nutrition advice. Combat Fat! doesn't require you to purchase special supplements. Food choices aren't limited to a zillion pounds of cabbage, and Combat Fat! will not require you to avoid a certain food group or nutrient. Results without effort aren't promised, and our program certainly is not revolutionary! On the contrary, Combat Fat! principles are based on decades of tested and retested scientific research.

At the core of Combat Fat! nutrition lies government recommendations based on the highest quality research to date.

Why are government recommendations more credible than most other recommendations? Motive is one reason. More than 50% of Americans over age 20 are overweight. The rate of diabetes is projected to double every 15 years. Healthcare costs, which the government has been trying desperately to contain, are soaring out of control. With these facts in mind, the government has an overwhelming reason to improve the health of our nation.

The quest for fame and fortune may be the driving force of other fitness promoters. "Lose 30 pounds in 30 days" sure makes a better headline than "Eat right and exercise more." Unfortunately, some research results are manipulated in order to benefit the pocketbooks of those funding the studies. The public is often misled because of their lack of expertise in the statistical skills needed to properly analyze these studies.

58

Preparing your kitchen to Combat Fat!

Now it's time to learn how to prepare your kitchen for Combat Fat! victory. **There are two main goals. The first goal is learning how to make healthy food choices. The second is to be able to easily identify correct portions to meet your fat loss goals.** Suggestions for stocking your pantry and cabinets along with your refrigerator and freezer are provided. Easy-to-follow menus, great recipes and multiple tips will guide you into eating healthy and controlling portions. The result—minimal casualties. Let the war begin!

Because life is not always predictable, there will be times when you feel ambushed and are unable to prepare the menu items suggested. With this in mind, we recommend that you keep both "quick to fix" and "grab and go" healthy foods in your home. Some suggestions include:

YOUR REFRIGERATOR

- Condiments including: a variety of mustards, catsup, reduced fat mayonnaise, reduced fat salad dressings, lemon juice and lime juice.
- Nonfat or 1% milk.
- Fresh fruit, fresh fruit, fresh fruit!
- Fresh vegetables including: romaine or leaf lettuce, tomatoes, onions, green peppers, carrots and sweet potatoes. Purchase ready-to- eat salad and pre-cut vegetables such as carrots, broccoli and cauliflower. If you float these pre-cut vegetables in water and cover, they will remain fresh and crisp for several days!
- Nonfat or lowfat yogurts.
- String cheese.
- Reduced fat shredded and sliced cheeses.
- Lower fat luncheon meats including: turkey breast, chicken breast and lean ham.

59

Stock up on spices!

In addition to salt and pepper, the following table provides guidance on which herbs and spices to keep on hand. It also indicates which foods their flavors would enhance. As you can see, the top 25 are extremely versatile.

ALLSPICE	Beef, poultry, fish, ham, soups, stews, vegetables, fruit.
BASIL	Beef, poultry, seafood, eggs, soups, stews, sauces, dips, salad dressings, vegetables, vinegar.
BAY LEAF	Beef, fish, beans, soups, stews, potatoes, rice, vinegar, marinates, gravies.
CAYENNE PEPPER	Beef, poultry, fish, soups, vegetables, pasta.
CHILI POWDER	Chili, soups, vegetables, beans, salads.
CHIVES	Soups, stews, sauces, dips, vegetables, salads, vinegars.
CILANTRO	Mexican and Asian dishes, curries, soups, stews, vegetables, fruit, desserts.
CINNAMON	Pork, poultry, lamb, breads, vegetables, pasta, rice, fruit, desserts, coffee.
CLOVES	Beef, pork, lamb, soups, stews, vegetables, desserts.
CUMIN	Mexican, Indian and Middle Eastern dishes, beef, lamb, pork, soups, stews, beans, chili, breads, sauces, dips, salad dressings, vinegar, desserts.
DILL	Beef, poultry, seafood, vegetables, salads and salad dressing, marinates, dips, sauces, beans, breads, soups, vinegar.
GINGER	Asian dishes, beef, poultry, fish, soups, stews, vegetables, breads, desserts.

60

GARLIC POWDER	Beef, poultry, soups, stews, beans, vegetables, salads and salad dressings, marinades, sauces, dips, pasta, breads, rice.
MARJORAM	Beef, poultry, seafood, soups, stews, sauces, dips, vegetables, breads, salads.
GROUND MUSTARD	Beef, poultry, fish, potatoes, marinades, sauces, cheese dips, salads, salad dressing.
NUTMEG	Beef, poultry, pork, soups, pasta, sauces. Vegetables, beans, fruit, desserts.
ONION POWDER	Beef, poultry, fish, soups, stews, beans, vegetables, breads, dips, sauces, marinades, salad dressings.
OREGANO	Beef, poultry, fish, pork, lamb, vegetables, sauces, salads, eggs, vinegar.
PAPRIKA	Beef, poultry, fish, soups, stews eggs, salads, salad dressing.
PARSLEY	Beef, poultry, fish, soups, stews, salads, vegetables, eggs, pasta, cheese, breads, sauces, grains, vinegar.
ROSEMARY	Beef, poultry, fish, lamb, vegetables, soups, stews, salads, potatoes, pasta, marinades, vinegar.
SAGE	Beef, poultry, pork, lamb, soups, stews, sauces, vegetables, pasta, casseroles, cheese, eggs, breads, grains, vinegar.
TARRAGON	Beef, poultry, fish, pasta, rice, grains, vegetables, marinades, vinegar.
THYME	Beef, poultry, fish, vegetables, soups, stews, salads, vinegar.

- Egg substitute.
- Fresh lemons and limes.

YOUR PANTRY

- Breakfast cereals that contain at least two grams of fiber per serving such as: all-bran, cracklin bran, frosted mini-wheats, Fruit & Fiber, raisin bran, shredded wheat and Wheaties.
- Instant hot cereals including oatmeal, grits and cream of wheat.
- Canned soups of the healthier variety such as Healthy Choice and Campbell's Healthy Request.
- Quick cooking white and brown rice.
- Tuna packed in water.
- Reduced fat tuna kits with crackers.
- Lower sodium spaghetti sauce such as Healthy Choice.
- A variety of pastas.
- Peanut butter (the freshly pressed variety has less saturated fat). Turn the container upside down after the first use then right side up after the next. This distributes the oil, making it easier to spread.
- Jelly.
- A variety of canned fruits in their own juice.
- Dried fruits.
- Nuts packaged in individual servings (for portion control).
- Pancake mix (buckwheat, if you can find it).
- Pancake syrup.
- Individual servings of applesauce in a variety of flavors.
- Vinegar (including balsamic).
- Canola and olive oils.
- Canned beans.

- Canned vegetables.
- Microwave popcorn of the healthier variety such as Orville Redenbacher's Smart Pop or Pop Secret's Light.
- Pretzels.
- Pizza sauce.

YOUR FREEZER

- Frozen whole grain waffles.
- Frozen pancakes.
- Frozen juice concentrates.
- A variety of frozen vegetables.
- Frozen berries.
- Frozen dinners of the healthier variety such as Healthy Choice, Lean Cuisine and Weight Watchers. Remember, your optimal sodium intake is no more than 2400 mg per day. This is 800 mg per meal. These brands usually meet those standards.
- Chicken breast, chicken breast, chicken breast!
- Whole wheat pizza crust.
- Veggie burgers.
- Frozen grilled fish fillets.
- Frozen fat-free chicken patties.
- A variety of whole grain breads. Breads freeze nicely and thaw quickly.

Navigating Past the Measuring Battles

Measuring every single morsel you put into your mouth gets frustrating. The Combat Fat! plan wants you to avoid this tedious task. Most menu items will be listed as "a bowl of" or "a handful of" rather than "2/3's of a cup of" the particular food. Obviously, if your handful is so large that you have food hanging between your fingers, the portion size is incorrect! Use the following to help you interpret the intended menu portions.

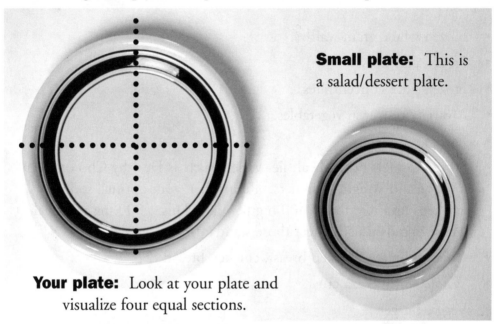

Small plate: This is a salad/dessert plate.

Your plate: Look at your plate and visualize four equal sections.

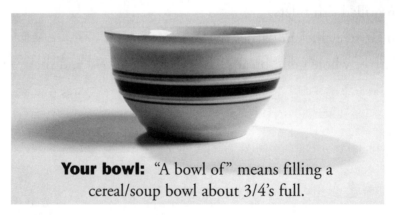

Your bowl: "A bowl of" means filling a cereal/soup bowl about 3/4's full.

64

:combat-fat.com www.combat-fat.com www.combat-fat.com www.combat-fat.com www.combat-fat.

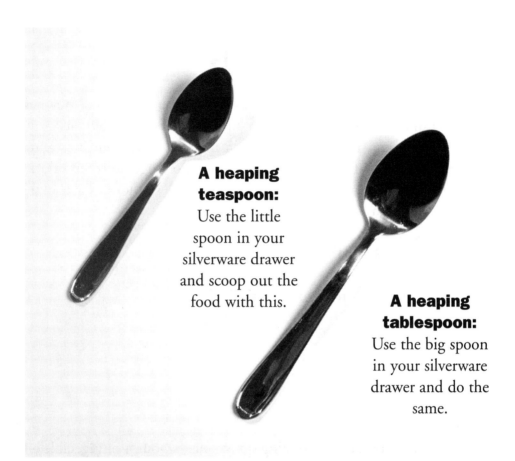

A heaping teaspoon: Use the little spoon in your silverware drawer and scoop out the food with this.

A heaping tablespoon: Use the big spoon in your silverware drawer and do the same.

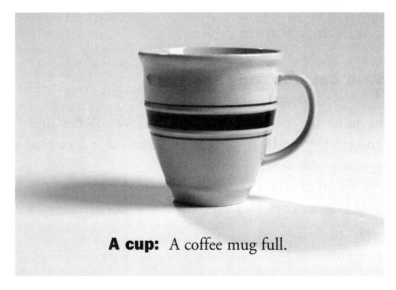

A cup: A coffee mug full.

Low-Calorie, Low-Fat
Cooking/Serving Methods

Cooking low-calorie, low-fat dishes may not take a long time, but best intentions can be lost with the addition of butter or other added fats at the table. It is important to learn how certain ingredients can add unwanted calories and fat to low-fat dishes—making them no longer lower in calories and lower in fat! The following list provides examples of lower fat-cooking methods and tips on how to serve your low-fat dishes.

Low-Fat Cooking Methods

These cooking methods tend to be lower in fat:
- Bake.

- Broil.

- Microwave.

- Roast—for vegetables and/or chicken without skin.

- Steam.

- Lightly stir-fry or sauté in cooking spray, small amounts of vegetable oil, or reduced sodium broth.

- Grill seafood, chicken or vegetables.

How To Save Calories and Fat

Look at the following examples for how to save calories and fat when preparing and serving foods. You might be surprised at how easy it is!

✔ Two tablespoons of butter on a baked potato can add an extra 200 calories and 22 grams of fat! However, ¼ cup salsa only adds 18 calories and no fat!

✔ Two tablespoons of regular clear Italian salad dressing will add an extra 136 calories and 14 grams of fat. Reduced fat Italian dressing only adds 30 calories and 2 grams of fat!

Try These Low-Fat Flavorings

- Herbs—oregano, basil, cilantro, thyme, parsley, sage, or rosemary.
- Spices—cinnamon, nutmeg, pepper, or paprika.
- Reduced-fat or fat-free salad dressing.
- Mustard.
- Catsup.
- Fat-free or reduced-fat mayonnaise.
- Fat-free or reduced-fat sour cream.
- Fat-free or reduced-fat yogurt.
- Reduced sodium soy sauce.
- Salsa.
- Lemon or lime juice.
- Vinegar.
- Horseradish.
- Fresh ginger.
- Sprinkle of butter flavor (not made with real butter).
- Red pepper flakes.
- Sprinkle of parmesan cheese (stronger flavor than most cheese).
- Sodium-free salt substitute.
- Jelly or fruit preserves on toast or bagels.

Alternatives to Eating High-Fat/High-Calorie Foods

These low-calorie alternatives should provide you with new ideas for old favorites.

Dairy Products

INSTEAD OF		USE THESE LOWER-FAT ALTERNATIVES
Evaporated whole milk.	☞	Evaporated fat-free (skim) or reduced-fat (2%) milk.
Whole milk.	☞	Low-fat (1%), reduced-fat (2%), or fat-free (skim) milk.
Ice cream.	☞	Sorbet, sherbet, low-fat or fat-free frozen yogurt, or ice milk (check label for calorie content).
Whipping cream.	☞	Imitation whipped cream (made with fat-free [skim] milk) or low-fat vanilla yogurt.
Sour cream.	☞	Plain low-fat yogurt.
Cream cheese.	☞	Neufchatel or "light" cream cheese or fat-free cream cheese.
Cheese.	☞	Reduced-calorie cheese, low-calorie processed cheeses, etc.
American cheese.	☞	Fat-free American cheese or other types of fat-free cheeses.
Regular (4%) cottage cheese.	☞	Low-fat (1%) or reduced-fat (2%) cottage cheese.
Whole milk mozzarella.	☞	Part-skim milk, low-moisture mozzarella cheese.
Whole milk ricotta.	☞	Part-skim milk ricotta cheese.
Coffee cream (1/2 and1/2) or nondairy creamer.	☞	Low-fat (1%) or reduced-fat (2%) milk or non-fat dry milk powder.

Cereals, Grains, and Pasta

INSTEAD OF		USE THESE LOWER-FAT ALTERNATIVES
Ramen noodles.	☞	Rice or noodles (spaghetti, macaroni, etc.).
Pasta with alfredo sauce.	☞	Pasta with marinara sauce.
Pasta with cheese sauce.	☞	Pasta with vegetables (primavera).
Granola.	☞	Bran flakes, crispy rice, etc.
	☞	Cooked grits or oatmeal.
	☞	Reduced-fat granola.

68

Meat, Fish, and Poultry

Coldcuts or lunch meats (bologna, salami, liverwurst, etc.).	☞	Low-fat coldcuts (95 to 97% fat-free lunch meats, low-fat pressed meats).
Hot dogs (regular).	☞	Lower-fat hot dogs.
Bacon or sausage.	☞	Canadian bacon or lean ham.
Regular ground beef.	☞	Extra lean ground beef such as ground round or ground turkey (read labels).
Chicken or turkey with skin; duck, or goose.	☞	Chicken or turkey without skin (white meat).
Oil-packed tuna.	☞	Water-packed tuna (rinse to reduce sodium content).
Beef (chuck, rib, brisket).	☞	Beef—round, loin (trimmed of external fat/ choose select grades).
Pork (spareribs, untrimmed loin).	☞	Pork tenderloin or trimmed, lean smoked ham.
Frozen breaded fish or fried fish.	☞	Fish or shellfish, unbreaded (fresh, frozen, canned in water).
Whole eggs.	☞	Egg whites or egg substitutes.
Frozen TV dinners (containing more than 13 grams of fat per serving).	☞	Frozen TV dinners (containing less than 13 grams of fat per serving and lower in sodium).
Chorizo sausage.	☞	Turkey sausage, drained well (read label).
	☞	Vegetarian sausage (made with tofu).

Baked Goods

Croissants, brioches, etc.	☞	Hard french rolls or soft brown 'n serve rolls.
Donuts, sweet rolls, muffins, scones, or pastries.	☞	English muffins, bagels, reduced-fat or fat-free muffins or scones.
Party crackers.	☞	Low-fat crackers (choose lower in sodium).
	☞	Saltine or soda crackers (choose lower in sodium).
Cake (pound, chocolate, yellow).	☞	Cake (angel food, white, gingerbread).
Cookies.	☞	Reduced-fat or fat-free cookies (graham crackers, ginger snaps, fig bars).

69

Snacks and Sweets

INSTEAD OF		USE THESE LOWER-FAT ALTERNATIVES
Nuts.	☞	Popcorn (air-popped or light microwave), fruits, vegetables.
Ice cream.	☞	Frozen yogurt, frozen fruit or chocolate pudding bars.
Custards or puddings (made with whole milk).	☞	Puddings (made with skim milk).

Fats, Oils, and Salad Dressings

INSTEAD OF		USE THESE LOWER-FAT ALTERNATIVES
Regular margarine or ter, butter.	☞	Light spread margarines, diet margarine, or whipped but-tub or squeeze bottle.
Regular mayonnaise.	☞	Light or diet mayonnaise or mustard.
Regular salad dressings.	☞	Reduced-calorie or fat-free salad dressings, lemon juice, or plain or herb flavored or wine vinegar.
Butter or margarine on toast or bread.	☞	Jelly, jam, or honey on bread or toast.
Oils, shortening, or lard.	☞	Nonstick cooking spray for stir-frying or sautéing.

Note: As a substitute for oil or butter, use applesauce or prune puree in baked goods

Miscellaneous

INSTEAD OF		USE THESE LOWER-FAT ALTERNATIVES
Canned cream soups.	☞	Canned broth-based soups.
Canned beans and franks.	☞	Canned baked beans in tomato sauce.
Gravy (homemade with fat and/or milk).	☞	Gravy mixes made with water or homemade with the fat skimmed off and fat-free milk.
Fudge sauce.	☞	Chocolate syrup.
Avocado on sandwiches.	☞	Cucumber slices or lettuce leaves.
Guacamole dip or refried beans with lard.	☞	Salsa.

70

Some suggested appliances for your Combat Fat! kitchen:

We use these daily to prepare healthy meals. These items save time and trouble and are available at most houseware stores.

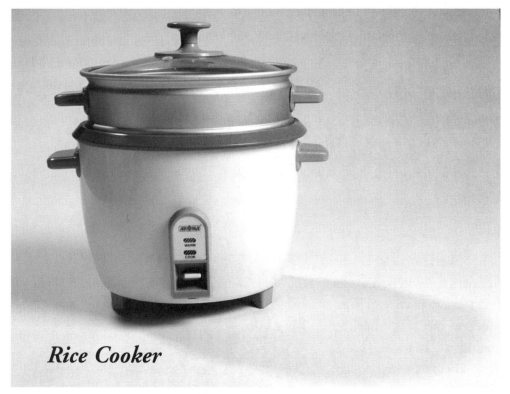

Rice Cooker

A rice cooker is a very versatile tool. Not only can you cook rice, you can steam vegetables, cook pasta, even prepare entire meals including beef, chicken or seafood. Cost is about $25.

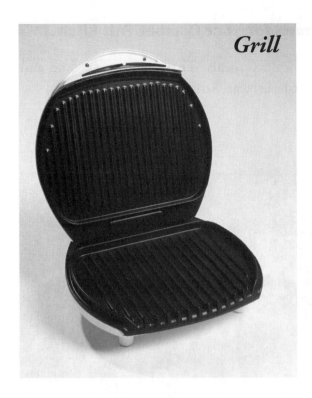

Grill

The countertop grill has evolved into a very reliable and even-cooking tool for your kitchen.

Meats, vegetables, and fish can be prepared creatively and tastily with a small amount of preparation. Cost ranges between $30 to $100 depending upon model and brand.

The workhorse of the modern kitchen, a microwave oven can produce a variety of healthy eating alternatives. From low-fat convenience foods, to popcorn, chicken breasts, steamed broccoli and other vegetables, sweet potatoes topped with tomato sauce and parmesan cheese…well, you get the idea! Cost under $100.

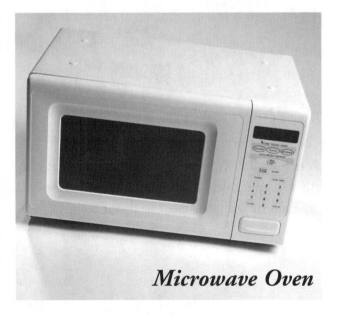

Microwave Oven

72

5
Combat Fat! Meal Plans

You've heard of painting by the numbers, no doubt. Well, here's our ultra-simple method for following a healthy, balanced diet. We call it "eating by the numbers."

On the following pages you will find meal selections for breakfast, lunch, a snack, and dinner. Each meal selection has been chosen for healthy ingredients and delicious preparation. Keep in mind, for the Combat Fat! meal plans to work their nutritional magic you need to respect the portion sizes that are presented—review the previous chapter if needed.

Note, too, that recipes are provided in the back of the book for those dishes which appear in **bold-faced type**. *More recipes are available on the combat-fat.com website.*

The meals selections have been developed for you by Laurie Cutlip, LN, RD, in accordance with the Dietary Guidelines for Americans *and the* Food Guide Pyramid.

Eat healthy and enjoy!

The Science Behind the Combat Fat! Meal Plans:

Separating food fact from food fantasy.

The meal plans are designed in accordance with the *Dietary Guidelines for Americans* and the Food Guide Pyramid. Each meal is packed with nutrient dense foods (foods having an abundance of vitamins, minerals and additional nutrients needed for good health compared with the calories they contain).

The menus are designed to provide about 1600 calories. Each meal is roughly 400 calories and snacks range from 50 to 150 calories. Proteins comprise 12% to 20% of total calories; carbohydrates, 55% to 60% and fats, 25% to 30%. Of course, when selecting recipes and planning menus we kept good nutrition in mind.

We also considered the ease in acquiring ingredients and the popularity of menu items. Every daily menu may not provide 100% of the recommended level of every single nutrient. Some days will contain a little more; some days, a little less. However, over the course of a few days, your nutrient intake will balance out and all of your needs will be met.

Recipes are provided for all items listed in bold print. They can be found in the back of the book.

The Combat Fat! Meal Plans

C'mon, admit it, we've all visited fast-food restaurants and have mastered the value meal system! If we want to choose the "#2" meal every time we drive up, we can. This is how the combat fat menu plan works. If a particular menu doesn't appeal to you, feel free to substitute another "value" meal, just don't super-size. Also remember that variety is the spice of life. Variety also ensures consumption of a diet containing adequate amounts of the nutrients required for optimal energy and health. Try to experiment with a number of these easy to prepare meals but let your taste buds navigate.

When reviewing your menus, you may want to plan a few days' worth of meals. This planning will allow you to use up ingredients you already have. For example, extra chicken left from dinner the night before can be used in a chicken salad recipe planned for lunch the following day. Vegetables required for tomorrow's dinner can be eaten raw at lunch today. This makes grocery shopping less cumbersome and your refrigerator won't become a science project.

At-a-Glance—

For breakfast choose 1 meal from the breakfast choices.
For lunch choose 1 meal from the lunch choices.
For dinner choose 1 meal from the dinner choices.
For snacks choose from the snack choices as required depending upon your calorie requirements.

COMBAT FAT! BREAKFAST CHOICES	COMBAT FAT! DINNER CHOICES
COMBAT FAT! LUNCH CHOICES	COMBAT FAT! SNACK CHOICES

COMBAT FAT! BREAKFAST CHOICES

BREAKFAST CHOICE #1

2 packets of instant oatmeal
1 small box of raisins
1 cup nonfat milk

BREAKFAST CHOICE #2

3 **Whole Wheat Pancakes** with
Strawberry Syrup
1 cup nonfat milk

BREAKFAST CHOICE #3

1 **Strawberry Orange Muffin**
1 banana
1 cup nonfat milk

BREAKFAST CHOICE #4

3 frozen pancakes with
2 heaping Tbsp of warm applesauce on top
1 cup nonfat milk

BREAKFAST CHOICE #5

1 **Blueberry Muffin**
1 small banana
1 cup nonfat milk

BREAKFAST CHOICE #6

2 slices **French Toast**
1 orange
1 slice Canadian bacon

BREAKFAST CHOICE #7

1 bowl high fiber cereal
1 cup nonfat milk
1 handful of nuts

BREAKFAST CHOICE #8

1/2 large bagel
2 heaping tsp of peanut butter
1 small box raisins
1 cup nonfat milk

COMBAT FAT! BREAKFAST CHOICES

BREAKFAST CHOICE #9

1 **Graham Cracker Muffin**
1 cup nonfat milk
1 small banana

BREAKFAST CHOICE #10

Greek Omelet
1/2 English muffin
1 tsp jam
1 cup berries

BREAKFAST CHOICE #11

2 slices whole-grain toast
2 heaping tsp jam
1/2 pt scrambled egg substitute
1/2 grapefruit

BREAKFAST CHOICE #12

1 nonfat yogurt mixed with
2 heaping tablespoons of
Grapenuts
1 cup grapefruit juice

BREAKFAST CHOICE #13

Potato and Cheese Omelet
1 slice whole wheat toast with
1 tsp butter
1/4 cantaloupe

COMBAT FAT! LUNCH CHOICES

LUNCH CHOICE #1

Veggie Pita Sandwich
1 apple
1 handful nuts

LUNCH CHOICE #2

Egg Salad Sandwich
raw cucumber wedges
1 apple

LUNCH CHOICE #3

1 **Sloppy Joe** sandwich
1 orange

LUNCH CHOICE #4

1 Turkey Roll-up
1 orange
1 handful of pretzels

LUNCH CHOICE #5

1 1/2 cups **Thai Pasta Salad**
1 pear

LUNCH CHOICE #6

1 **Strawberry Orange Muffin**
1 apple
1 nonfat, no sugar added yogurt

COMBAT FAT! LUNCH CHOICES

LUNCH CHOICE #7

1 cup **Cheese Ravioli Soup**
4 saltines
1 apple

LUNCH CHOICE #8

Lemony Chickpea Dip Pita
sandwich
1 orange

LUNCH CHOICE #9

1 bowl **Stovetop Lentil Casserole**
4 saltines
1 plum

LUNCH CHOICE #10

1 plate **Spinach Salad**
1 handful grapes
1/2 small whole grain bagel
1 tsp butter

LUNCH CHOICE #11

1 cup **Chunk Beef & Vegetable Soup**
1/2 bagel
1 tsp butter

LUNCH CHOICE #12

Chicken Salad Sandwich
1 cup grapes
1 handful raw baby carrots

79

COMBAT FAT! LUNCH CHOICES

LUNCH CHOICE #13

1 cup **Chicken and Sundried Tomato Pasta Salad**
1 cup nonfat milk
1 orange

LUNCH CHOICE #14

1 cup **Spunky Chili**
2 saltines
2 raw apricots

LUNCH CHOICE #15

1 **Better than Pizza Potato**
1 plum

LUNCH CHOICE #16

1 nonfat yogurt
1 cup strawberries

LUNCH CHOICE #17

1 **Brunch Wrap**
1 handful raw baby carrots
1 cup nonfat milk

LUNCH CHOICE #18

1 small plate **Waldorf Salad**
4 saltines

COMBAT FAT! LUNCH CHOICES

LUNCH CHOICE #19

2 slices rye bread
3 slices deli turkey breast
1 tbsp lowfat mayo
lettuce and tomato
1 handful baked chips
1 handful blueberries

LUNCH CHOICE #20

2 slices whole grain bread
2 slices deli roast beef
1 tbsp light mayo
lettuce and tomato
1 pear

LUNCH CHOICE #21

1 small bagel with
2 slices lean ham,
1 slice lowfat cheese and
Dijon mustard
1 handful cherry tomatoes
1 peach

LUNCH CHOICE #22

2 slices whole grain bread
2 deli slices lean ham
1 slice lowfat cheese
1 tbsp Dijon mustard
1 handful baked chips
1 handful fresh cherries

COMBAT FAT! DINNER CHOICES

DINNER CHOICE #1

1 piece **Krispy Chicken**
1/4 plate **Smashed Potatoes**
1/2 plate nutty balsamic green beans
1 individual container applesauce

DINNER CHOICE #2

1 piece **Southwestern Pork Tenderloin**
1 ear corn
1/2 plate vegetable salad
2 shakes lowfat salad dressing

DINNER CHOICE #3

1/4 plate **Teriyaki Steak Fingers**
1/4 plate **Smashed Potatoes**
1 small vegetable salad
2 shakes lowfat salad dressing

DINNER CHOICE #4

1 piece **Baked Chicken Siciliano**
1/4 plate cooked rotini pasta with tomato sauce
1 small vegetable salad
2 shakes lowfat salad dressing

DINNER CHOICE #5

1 bowl **Pasta Primavera**
1 small vegetable salad
2 shakes lowfat dressing
1 slice Italian bread

DINNER CHOICE #6

1/4 plate **Chicken Tenders**
1/4 plate **Dash Slaw**
1 cup strawberries

82

COMBAT FAT! DINNER CHOICES

DINNER CHOICE #7

1 piece **Buttery Almond Fish**
1/4 plate brown rice
1/2 plate broccoli
1 cup nonfat milk

DINNER CHOICE #8

1/4 plate baked ham
1/4 plate brown rice
1/4 plate **Cheesy Broccoli Gratin**
1 kiwi

DINNER CHOICE #9

1 piece **Grilled Marinated Salmon**
1/4 plate Rice Pilaf
1/2 plate **Spinach Salad**

DINNER CHOICE #10

3/4 cup **Barbeque Pork Sandwich**
1 whole grain hamburger bun
1 cup Dash Slaw
1 small watermelon wedge

DINNER CHOICE #11

1 bowl **Stovetop Lentil Casserole**
1 small plate of vegetable salad
2 shakes lowfat salad dressing
1 small dinner roll
1 tsp butter

DINNER CHOICE #12

1 1/2 cups **Thai Pasta Salad**
1 small plate mixed berries
1 small dinner roll
1 tsp butter

COMBAT FAT! DINNER CHOICES

DINNER CHOICE #13

1 bowl **Spunky Chili**
4 saltines
1 small plate vegetable salad
2 shakes lowfat salad dressing

DINNER CHOICE #14

1/2 plate **Pot Roast and Vegetables**
1/2 plate **Spinach Salad**
1 individual container applesauce

DINNER CHOICE #15

1 **Kielbasa on a Skewer**
1 small baked sweet potato sprayed with nonfat butter spray and sprinkled with cinnamon
1 small salad
2 shakes nonfat salad dressing

DINNER CHOICE #16

1 piece **Grilled Curried Tofu**
1/2 plate grilled eggplant
1/4 plate cooked lentils

DINNER CHOICE #17

1 bowl **Cheese Ravioli Soup**
1 small vegetable salad
2 shakes lowfat salad dressing
1 small dinner roll
1 tsp butter

DINNER CHOICE #18

1 **Sloppy Joe** sandwich
1/4 plate cooked corn
1/2 plate vegetable salad
2 shakes lowfat salad dressing

COMBAT FAT! DINNER CHOICES

DINNER CHOICE #19

1 piece **Chicken Del Jardin**
1/4 plate couscous
1/4 plate **Roasted Carrots with Lime**

DINNER CHOICE #20

1/2 plate **Spaghetti Squash Pomodoro**
1/2 plate **Spinach Salad**
1 small dinner roll
1 tsp butter

DINNER CHOICE #21

1 piece **Chicken Cacciatore**
1/4 plate cooked bowtie pasta with sauce
1 small salad
2 shakes lowfat salad dressing

DINNER CHOICE #22

1 bowl **Chunk Beef and Vegetable Soup**
1 small vegetable salad
2 shakes lowfat salad dressing
1 small dinner roll
1 tsp butter

DINNER CHOICE #23

1 piece **Citrus Orange Roughy**
1/4 plate brown rice
1/4 plate peas
1/4 of a cantaloupe

DINNER CHOICE #24

1 **Oaty Hamburger**
1 hamburger bun
1 small salad
2 shakes lowfat salad dressing

85

COMBAT FAT! DINNER CHOICES

DINNER CHOICE #25

1 **Pork Chop Dijon**
1/2 small sweet potato
1/2 plate steamed asparagus,
sprinkled with lime juice

86

.combat-fat.com www.combat-fat.com www.combat-fat.com www.combat-fat.com www.combat-fat.

COMBAT FAT! DINNER CHOICES

IF TIME IS LIMITED CONSIDER THE FOLLOWING MENUS

DINNER CHOICE #1

1 can Healthy Choice Soup
1 small roll
1 tsp butter

DINNER CHOICE #2

1 lowfat hotdog
1 hotdog bun
1 handful lowfat chips
1/4 plate baked beans

DINNER CHOICE #3

1 Lean Cuisine Frozen dinner
1/2 grapefruit
1 cup nonfat milk

DINNER CHOICE #4

1 tuna and cracker kit
1 bowl of grapes

DINNER CHOICE #5

1 Weight Watchers Frozen
Dinner
1 small roll
1 tsp butter

COMBAT FAT! SNACK CHOICES

Pick 3 snack servings per day to achieve your nutrition goal of approximately 1600 calories per day.

● ● ● ● ● ● ● ●

Note: You can adjust your calorie intake by adding/subtracting snacks each day.

If, for example, after three weeks of following the plan, you feel that you are not losing enough fat, simply <u>reduce</u> the number of snack portions.

Conversely, you can <u>add</u> snack portions if you feel you are losing too much fat too quickly.

Keep in mind that each snack provides about 50 - 150 calories per portion.

COMBAT FAT! SNACK CHOICES

SNACK CHOICE #1
1 large handful of grapes

SNACK CHOICE #2
1 cup of juice

SNACK CHOICE #3
1 container of nonfat, no sugar added fruited yogurt

SNACK CHOICE #4
1/2 bag light microwave popcorn

SNACK CHOICE #5
1 handful of baked tortillas with salsa

SNACK CHOICE #6
1 slice string cheese with 3 crackers

SNACK CHOICE #7
1 **Strawberry Orange Muffin**

SNACK CHOICE #7
1 cup fresh berries

SNACK CHOICE #8
2 large graham crackers

SNACK CHOICE #9
1/2 baked potato with salsa

SNACK CHOICES

SNACK CHOICE #10

2 large popcorn or rice cakes

SNACK CHOICE #11

6-8 whole grain crackers

SNACK CHOICE #12

1 handful of steamed shrimp sprinkled with lemon juice and/or Old Bay seasoning

SNACK CHOICE #13

1 handful raw veggies dipped in **Lemony Chickpea Dip Pita** filling.

SNACK CHOICE #14

2 handfuls raw veggies with 2 shakes of reduced fat salad dressing to dip

SNACK CHOICE #15

1 slice of lowfat cheese or luncheon meat cut up on top of leftover salad with 2 shakes of reduced fat salad dressing

SNACK CHOICE #16

1/2 prepared **Grilled Pineapple Slices**

SNACK CHOICE #17

1 tsp peanut butter and 3 crackers

90

SNACK CHOICES

SNACK CHOICE #18

1 lowfat bran muffin

SNACK CHOICE #19

1 cup of milk

SNACK CHOICE #20

1 cup soup

SNACK CHOICE #21

1 frozen fruit juice bar

SNACK CHOICE #22

1 handful any variety of Teddy Grahams

SNACK CHOICE #23

1 pancake with a squeeze of light syrup

SNACK CHOICE #24

1 piece fresh fruit

SNACK CHOICE #25

1 handful dried fruit

SNACK CHOICE #26

1 handful of pretzels

SNACK CHOICE #27

1/2 small bagel with jam

COMBAT FAT RECIPES

BAKED CHICKEN SICILIANO

1 15 ounce can tomato sauce
4 tsp Mrs. Dash Classic Italiano Blend, divided
1/2 cup grated Parmesan cheese, divided
8 boneless, skinless chicken breasts

Preheat oven to 400 degrees.
Combine tomato sauce, 3 tsp Mrs. Dash and 1/2 cup cheese in bowl.
Coat chicken with mixture.
Place chicken in baking dish.
Sprinkle on remaining cheese and Mrs. Dash.
Bake for 40 minutes.
MAKES 8 SERVINGS

BARBEQUE PORK

1 1/4 pounds pork shoulder, boneless
1 diced onion
2 tbsp minced garlic
2 tbsp sugar
1/2 tsp Dijon mustard
1 cup catsup
3 tbsp Worcestershire sauce.

Cut pork crosswise into 1/4 inch slices.
Combine all ingredients except pork in small bowl.
Mix well.
Add pork and mixture to slow cooker.
Cook on low for 6 hours or until tender
MAKES 4 SERVINGS

BETTER THAN PIZZA POTATOES

4 Medium Potatoes, baked
1/4 tsp oregano
1/4 cup chopped red and green bell peppers
4 tsp Molly McButter Natural Butter Flavor Sprinkles
4 tbsp shredded lowfat Mozzarella cheese
1/4 cup canned diced tomatoes, drained
Mrs. Dash Extra Spicy Blend to taste

92

Preheat oven to 350 degrees
Slice open tops of potato, leaving 1/4 inch of skin on each side.
Scoop out potato from shells.
Blend with potato all ingredients except cheese and Mrs. Dash.
Spoon mixture into shells and top with cheese.
Bake until well heated (about 10 minutes).
These can also be heated in a microwave (2 to 3) minutes.
Sprinkle with Mrs. Dash to taste and serve
MAKES 4 SERVINGS

BLUEBERRY MUFFINS

2 cups flour
1/3 cup granulated sugar
1 tsp baking powder
1 tsp baking soda
1/4 cup orange juice
2 tbsp canola oil
1 tsp vanilla extract
8 ounce container of vanilla yogurt (or blueberry)
1 egg
1 cup blueberries (frozen can be used if thawed).

Preheat oven to 400 degrees.
Combine dry ingredients in a large bowl.
Mix remaining ingredients in a separate bowl.
Spoon batter into lined muffin tin
Sprinkle with a small amount of sugar, if desired
Bake 17 to 19 minutes.
MAKES 12 MUFFINS

BRUNCH WRAPS

10 ounce package of frozen, chopped spinach, thawed and drained
1/2 cup nonfat sour cream
2 tsp Mrs. Dash Italiano Blend
4 large flour tortillas
2 cups chopped salad mix
1 cup chopped tomatoes
1 cup cooked, diced chicken
1/4 cup chopped scallions
1/4 cup shredded lowfat mozzarella cheese

Combine spinach, sour cream and Mrs. Dash in small bowl.
Mix well.
Spread spinach mix onto tortillas (about 1/4 cup for each) covering entire tortilla.

93

Top each tortilla with 1/4 of the remaining ingredients
Fold tortilla top and bottom over filling, then roll sides to form a tightly rolled sandwich.
Wrap in plastic wrap and refrigerate at least 2 hours.
Serve chilled.
MAKES 4 SERVINGS.

BUTTERY ALMOND FISH

1 1/2 tbsp Molly Mc Butter Natural Butter Flavor Sprinkles
1 1/2 tsp Mrs. Dash Lemon Pepper Blend
1/2 tsp lime juice
1/2 tsp water
1/2 tsp honey
8 ounces boneless, white fish fillets
1 1/2 tbsp sliced toasted almonds

Combine first 5 ingredients in a bowl and mix well.
Broil fish 6 to 8 inches from heat for 5 minutes, turning once.
Spread mixture over fish.
Broil another 4 to 5 minutes.
Sprinkle with almonds and serve.
MAKES 2 SERVINGS

CHEESY BROCCOLI GRATIN

4 1/2 cups day old white bread, crusts removed, cut into 1/2 inch cubes
6 tbsp Molly Mc Butter Natural Cheese Flavor Sprinkles, divided
1 tsp Mrs. Dash Extra Spicy Blend
1 tsp prepared yellow mustard
2 cups nonfat milk
20 ounces of frozen broccoli spears, thawed

Preheat oven to 400 degrees.
Place bread in large bowl.
Sprinkle on all of Mrs. Dash and 4 tbsp of Molly Mc Butter.
Combine mustard and milk in small bowl.
Pour over bread mixture and let sit 5 minutes.
Coat 13x9 inch baking dish with non-stick spray.
Arrange broccoli in dish.
Evenly pour bread mixture over broccoli.
Sprinkle with remaining Molly Mc Butter
Bake until golden brown and bubbly (30-40 minutes).
MAKES 8 SERVINGS

94

Helpful Hints

1. Prepare a batch of muffins from the recipe section. Individually freeze those you don't intend to eat that day. They can be taken out at a later date and rapidly thawed on the counter, or in the microwave. This will prevent you from having "just one more," and makes for a quick snack or breakfast.

2. If you are not particularly hungry, save part of your meal for a snack later in the day.

3. When choosing raw vegetables for snacks, be adventurous. Raw pepper slices, cucumber wedges, radishes, zucchini slices and grape tomatoes all will give your taste buds a welcome change to the usual carrot and celery slices.

4. For a delicious frozen dessert, freeze your nonfat or lowfat yogurt. Stir the yogurt prior to freezing if the fruit is on the bottom.

5. When choosing nuts, don't forget about soy nuts. These delicious crunchy nuts may help reduce cholesterol as well as have other health benefits. They are usually available on a rack in the produce section of your grocery store.

6. Make your own combat fat frozen dinners using leftovers from your value meal. Plate and freeze these meals prior to dining and you won't be tempted to have "seconds".

7. Purchase inexpensive compartmentalized storage containers. This will make plating leftovers for you own frozen dinners a breeze!

8. To prevent sandwiches from getting soggy, use toasted bread.

9. When choosing snacks, keep in mind adults should have a minimum of 2 cups of milk daily to meet their calcium requirements.

10. When choosing lowfat salad dressing, check the labels for calories. Try to select those with fewer than 40 calories per serving.

CHEESE RAVIOLI SOUP

4 cans (20 ounces each) chicken broth
16 ounce package of frozen red pepper stir-fry
4 tbsp Mrs. Dash Classic Italiano Blend
13 ounce package frozen mini cheese ravioli

Combine broth, stir-fry and Mrs. Dash in medium saucepan.
Bring to a boil.
Add ravioli.
Simmer 15 to 20 minutes.
Serve.
MAKES 6 SERVINGS

CHICKEN AND SUN DRIED TOMATO PASTA SALAD

2 cups uncooked bow tie pasta
14 ounce can of artichoke hearts, drained and chopped
1 1/2 cups chopped, cooked chicken
2 cups cooked broccoli florets
1/2 cup sun dried tomato strips with oil
2 tbsp balsamic vinegar
4 tsp Mrs. Dash Classic Italiano Blend

Cook pasta as directed on package.
Combine all ingredients with drained pasta and mix well.
Serve chilled.
MAKES 6 SERVINGS

CHICKEN CACCIATORE

2-tsp olive oil
6 boneless, skinless chicken breasts
3/4 cup chopped green bell pepper
3/4 cup sliced mushrooms
14.5 ounce can of pasta ready tomatoes, undrained
2 tbsp parsley
1 1/2 tbsp Mrs. Dash Classic Italiano Blend

Heat olive oil in large skillet over medium heat
Add chicken and brown.
Add remaining ingredients.
Simmer uncovered for 10-12 minutes.
MAKES 6 SERVINGS

96

CHICKEN DEL JARDIN

4 boneless, skinless chicken breasts
2 tsp Mrs. Dash Extra Spicy Seasoning Blend
4 small zucchini, halved and sliced to 1/4 inch thick
8-ounce can of no-salt added corn
2/3,s cup mild picante sauce

Coat skillet with non-stick spray.
Warm skillet over medium heat.
Pound chicken to 1/4 inch thickness.
Add chicken to hot skillet and cook 2 minutes.
Turn and sprinkle each piece with Mrs. Dash.
Cook another minute or so until thoroughly cooked.
Remove chicken and cover it to keep it warm.
Add all other ingredients to skillet.
Simmer until zucchini is tender (about 5 minutes) stirring occasionally.
Top chicken with sauce and serve.
MAKES 4 SERVINGS.

CHICKEN SALAD SANDWICH

1 leftover cooked chicken breast from any recipe
1/4 tsp Italian seasoning
1 chopped celery stalk
1 chopped scallion
1 tbsp lemon juice
1/4 cup lowfat mayonnaise
5 seedless grapes, each cut into 4 pieces

Finely cube chicken
Mix in remaining ingredients
Serve salad, topped with lettuce and tomato, between 2 slices of toasted whole grain bread
MAKES 2 SERVINGS

DASH SLAW

4 cups thinly shredded cabbage
1/4 cup light mayonnaise
1/4 cup lowfat sour cream
1 tbsp lemon juice
2 tsp Mrs.Dash Tomato Basil Garlic

Combine all ingredients except cabbage in a bowl.
Pour over cabbage and mix well.
Refrigerate at least 2 hours.
MAKES 4 SERVINGS

97

Your New Friend—Balsamic Vinegar

Balsamic vinegar is a wonderful condiment to have in your Combat Fat! kitchen. Flavorful, versatile, sweet yet tangy, it is equally at home with chicken, beef, vegetables, salads, and more. A simple grilled chicken breast served over a mixed salad and drizzled with balsamic vinegar makes a delightful lunch.

Balsamic vinegars are originally from the area around Modena in central Italy and are made from trebbiano grapes and are then put through a unique aging process, being stored in a succession of different kinds of wooden barrels until they are at their peak.

Vinegar and boiled wine have been a universal feature of Italian cuisine since ancient Roman times, and it is from boiled wine that balsamic vinegar initially originated.

The term "balsamic" derives from the old tradition of using this vinegar as a medicine and as a remedy for stomachache; during the plague in the XVII century, for example, it was used as a disinfectant.

Special vinegars have been made in the area around Modena for centuries, and the environmental conditions (soil and climate) and the local grapes are ideal.

The "secret of vinegar-making" was jealously guarded from generation to generation, to prevent a reduction in the status of this highly prized product, used above all for celebrations, gifts and special occasions.

Balsamic vinegar can be purchased at your local grocery store.

EGG SALAD SANDWICH

1/2 cup egg substitute
1/4 cup lowfat mayonnaise
1 tbsp Dijon mustard
3 hard cooked egg whites
2 chopped scallions
2 chopped celery stalks
1/4 tsp Tabasco sauce

Coat skillet with non-stick spray
Pour in egg substitute
Cook covered over medium heat (do not scramble during cooking)
Chop cooked egg substitute and egg whites
In bowl mix all ingredients
Serve salad, topped with lettuce and tomato, on 2 slices of toasted whole grain bread
MAKES 2 SERVINGS

CHICKEN TENDERS

1 pound chicken tenders or strips
1/2 cup catsup
1 1/2 tsp Mrs. Dash Original Seasoning
1 1/2 tsp Mrs. Dash Extra Spicy Seasoning
2 tbsp brown sugar
1 tbsp olive oil

Combine all ingredients except chicken in a small bowl.
Let stand for at least 1 hour.
Remove chicken from refrigerator.
Coat chicken with sauce mix.
Broil for 10 to 12 minutes, turning once.
MAKES 4 SERVINGS

CHUNK BEEF AND VEGETABLE SOUP

1 tbsp canola oil
1 1/4 pounds beef shank crosscuts
2 quarts water
1 cup diced celery
1/2 cup chopped onion
10 ounce package frozen mixed vegetables
1 cup salt-free canned tomatoes, chopped
6 ounces can salt-free tomato paste
1 tbsp sugar
2 1/2 tsp Mrs. Dash All-Purpose Original Blend
2 tsp vinegar

1/4 cup cold water
2 tbsp cornstarch

Heat oil in large saucepan.
Add beef and brown over medium heat
Add water, celery and onion to pot.
Bring to boil, reduce heat and simmer for 2 hours.
Remove shanks and cool.
Stir in remaining ingredients, (except water, meat and cornstarch)
Simmer for 1 hour.
Remove meat from shanks and cut into small chunks.
Return cut meat to pot.
Mix cold water and cornstarch in small bowl until smooth.
Add to pot and stir until slightly thickened.
MAKES 8 SERVINGS

CITRUS ORANGE ROUGHY

1 pound orange roughly fillets
1 tbsp Mrs. Dash Tomato Basil Garlic
2 slices fresh orange
2 slices fresh lemon
2 slices fresh lime

Preheat oven to 350 degrees.
Arrange fish in baking dish.
Sprinkle with Mrs. Dash and top with fruit slices.
Bake 15-20 minutes (until fish is opaque and easily flakes with fork).
MAKES 4 SERVINGS

FRENCH TOAST

8 slices whole grain bread
1/2 carton egg substitute
1 whole egg
2 tbsp nonfat milk
1/2 tsp vanilla
1/4 tsp cinnamon

Combine all ingredients except bread in a shallow dish
Whisk until well blended
Soak bread in mixture, turning once
Coat skillet with non-stick spray
Cook until brown over medium heat turning once
MAKES 8 SERVINGS

100

Your New Friend—The Granny Smith Apple

For years I avoided eating apples. For some reason, the skin made my gums itch! This is true. Cherries were even worse. My lips itched, my entire mouth itched.

Then one day recently, a friend introduced me to the Granny Smith. Hesitant at first, I nibbled a bit off and found to my surprise…no itchy teeth. I took another bite, then another. Delightful. Succulent. Tangy. Juicy. These were the thoughts that drove through my senses!

Since then, I have sought out these delicious bright green highly polished apples whenever they are available—for many good reasons—not just taste!

Apples are high in dietary fiber and a medium apple contains just 80 fat-free calories. Plus apples come in their own biodegradable packaging, unlike most other snacks.

Additionally, there is overwhelming scientific research proving apples promote good health. Apples contain numerous vitamins, minerals, and nutrients that are enormously beneficial. Some of the latest research indicates that eating apples every day may help prevent illnesses such as cancer and heart disease.

So the old adage "an apple a day keeps the doctor away" might just be true!

GRAHAM CRACKER MUFFINS

3 cups crushed graham crackers (any flavor)
1/4 cup sugar
2 tsp baking powder
1 cup nonfat milk
1/4 cup egg substitute
1 tbsp vanilla extract
Preheat oven to 400 degrees
Combine dry ingredients in a large bowl
Add wet ingredients and stir.
Spoon batter into lined muffin tin
Bake 14-16 minutes
MAKES 8 MUFFINS

GREEK OMELET

1 egg
3/4 cup egg substitute
1/2 cup cooked, warm, chopped spinach (microwave)
1/4 cup finely chopped, cooked onion (microwave until soft)
1 oz crumbled feta cheese
1-tsp butter

Mix egg and egg substitute
Melt butter in non-stick skillet
Partially cook eggs in skillet over medium heat
Turn eggs and sprinkle on cheese and vegetables
Finish cooking omelet.
Fold over and serve.
MAKES 2 SERVINGS

GRILLED EGGPLANT WEDGES

1 eggplant cut into16 wedges
1/4 cup olive oil
1 1/2 tsp garlic powder

Preheat George Foreman grill
Combine garlic and olive oil in small bowl
Brush mixture onto wedges.
Grill 2 to 3 minutes.
MAKES 8 SERVINGS

GRILLED PINEAPPLE SLICES

1 can (about 15 ounces) sliced pineapple in its own juice
1 tbsp brown sugar

102

I Can't Believe It's Not Butter spray

Preheat George Foreman Grill
Drain pineapple and coat each slice with 1 spray of butter spray
Sprinkle with sugar and grill about 1 minute.
MAKES 2 SERVINGS

GRILLED CURRIED TOFU

1 package of extra firm tofu, well drained
2 tbsp canola oil
3 tbsp cumin
1 tbsp chili powder
1 tbsp chopped onion
1 tbsp sugar
1/4 cup of lemon juice

Slice tofu into 4's.
Mix all ingredients except tofu in a shallow bowl to make marinate.
Marinate for at least 1 hour in the refrigerator, turning once.
Preheat George Foreman grill.
Grill 2 to 3 minutes.
MAKES 4 SERVINGS

GRILLED MARINATED SALMON

4 salmon fillets (about 4 ounces each)
1/4 cup lite soy sauce
1/2 cup sweet wine
2 tbsp lime juice
3 tbsp chopped scallions

Combine all liquid ingredients in shallow dish.
Add salmon and marinate in refrigerator for at least 2 hours.
Preheat grill.
Grill fish for 2 minutes.
Turn and grill another 1 to 2 minutes.
Sprinkle with scallions and serve.
MAKES 4 SERVINGS

KIELBASA ON A SKEWER

1 zucchini cut into 1-inch chunks
1 onion cut into I inch chunks
1 red pepper, cored and cut into 1 inch chunks
1 cup reduced fat Italian salad dressing
1 pound Healthy Choice Kielbasa cut into 1-inch chunks

103

6 wooden skewers

Mix vegetables and Italian dressing.
Soak skewers in water.
Cover and refrigerate for at least 2 hours.
Preheat grill.
Thread 1 chunk of each vegetable and 1then 1 chunk of kielbasa. Repeat.
Grill until vegetables are tender (about 8 minutes)
MAKES 6 SERVINGS

KRISPY CHICKEN

4 boneless, skinless chicken breasts
11/2 cups crushed unsweetened bran cereal
1/4 cup nonfat milk
1 tbsp canola or olive oil
11/2 tsp minced garlic
11/2-tsp paprika

Preheat oven to 350 degrees
In shallow dish combine all dry ingredients
Whisk oil into milk
Brush both sides of chicken with milk mixture
Coat with dry mixture
Bake for 18 minutes
Turn and bake another 10 minutes or until done.
MAKES 4 SERVINGS

LEMONY CHICKPEA DIP PITA SANDWICH

15 ounce can garbanzo beans, rinsed and drained
1/4 cup water
1/2 cup nonfat, plain yogurt
1 tbsp Mrs. Dash Lemon Pepper Blend
1/4 cup shredded carrots
3 tbsp chopped scallions
1 large romaine lettuce leaf
1/2 whole wheat pita bread

Combine first 4 ingredients, puree until smooth.
Stir in scallions and carrots.
Line pita with lettuce.
Fill pita with 3 heaping tbsp of puree mixture.
MAKES 5 SERVINGS

104

Your New Friend—Tofu

I know what you're thinking: "Ok, they're going to make me eat tofu. I knew it!"

Stop right there. We are not going to make you do anything you don't want to do. But keep in mind that tofu, available in the fresh vegetable section of most supermarkets, is an excellent alternative to chicken, fish, or beef in many dishes.

A staple in Asia for 2,000 years, tofu is known for its extraordinary nutritional benefits, as well as its versatility. It is high in protein and calcium, low in calories and is cholesterol-free.

Tofu is made with soy. Soy is the only legume with complete protein, containing all eight essential amino acids. An eight-ounce serving of tofu can provide an adult male with about 27 percent of his daily protein requirement. Tofu contains no cholesterol and very little sodium, but has as much calcium as milk, and has, serving for serving, less than half the fat of most other protein sources. Tofu is also an important source of vitamins and minerals.

In equal servings, tofu has 25-50 percent less calories than beef, and 40 percent less calories than eggs. A four-ounce serving of extra firm tofu has less than 120 calories, compared to 455 calories for the same portion of cheddar cheese.

NUTTY BALSAMIC GREEN BEANS

1# green beans trimmed and washed
1/8 cup toasted chopped walnuts
1/4 cup chopped Spanish onion
1/4 cup broth (any variety)
2 tbsp balsamic vinegar

Steam beans until bright green and drain.
Toast nuts in non-stick skillet until brown (about 3 minutes).
Cook onion in non-stick skillet until tender (about 3 minutes)
Combine all of the ingredients except the nuts to the skillet and simmer until most of the liquid has evaporated.
Toss with nuts and serve
MAKES 4 SERVINGS

Your New Friend — The Lemon

The lemon—and its kissing cousin, the lime—provide a wonderful zest to any dish you prepare. Squeezed on a salad, sliced and sautéed with a chicken breast, served on the side with fish...there are innumerable ways to cook with these citrus fruits!

Keep a lemon in the fridge, or if unavailable, a squeeze bottle of Real-Lemon or Real-Lime juice. Though reconstituted lemon and lime juice can't replace fresh squeezed, they do provide a reliable source of this tasty addition!

106

OATY HAMBURGERS

1/2 pound extra lean hamburger meat
1 1/2 cup uncooked oatmeal
1/2 small onion, chopped
1-cup marinara sauce

Preheat grill.
Combine all ingredients and mix well.
Shape mixture into 8 burgers.
Grill to your desired doneness.
MAKES 6 BURGERS

PASTA PRIMAVERA

1 package angel hair pasta
2 tbsp olive oil
2 tbsp minced garlic
1/2 cup chopped onion
4 chopped tomatoes
1 cup mushroom slices
1 cup thin zucchini slices
2 tbsp grated Parmesan cheese

Cook pasta according to package directions.
Sauté garlic and onion in olive oil for 1 minute.
Add zucchini and sauté another minute.
Add tomatoes and mushrooms.
Cook until heated through.
Top pasta with mixture, sprinkle with cheese and serve.
MAKES 8 SERVINGS

PORK CHOPS DIJON

2 pork loin chops
1/2 tsp low-sodium chicken broth
2 tbsp honey
4 tsp Dijon mustard
1 tbsp Mrs. Dash Garlic & Herb Blend

Preheat oven to 350 degrees.
Combine all ingredients, except pork chops, in baking dish.
Mix well.
Add pork chops.
Bake, covered 25 minutes.
Uncover and cook 10 more minutes.
MAKES 2 SERVINGS

PORK TENDERLOIN IN CREAM SAUCE

1 1/2 pounds pork tenderloin
1 can sliced mushrooms, drained
2 cans cream of mushroom sauce
1 tsp black pepper

Put pork in slow cooker.
Sprinkle pepper on top.
Pour in mushrooms and soup.
Cook on low for 8 hours.
MAKES 6 SERVINGS

POTATO AND CHEESE OMELET

1 egg
3/4 cup egg substitute
3/4 cup diced cooked warm potatoes
3/4 cup lowfat cheese
1 tsp butter

Mix egg and egg substitute
Melt butter in non-stick skillet
Partially cook eggs in skillet over medium heat
Turn eggs and sprinkle on cheese and potatoes.
Finish cooking omelet.
Fold over and serve.
MAKES 2 SERVINGS

POT ROAST AND VEGETABLES

6 small potatoes, peeled and quartered
1 small bag baby carrots
1 large onion, peeled and sliced
3 pounds beef sirloin
2 tbsp minced garlic
1 tsp pepper
1 tsp paprika
1/4 cup Worcestershire sauce
1 can low salt beef broth
1 bay leaf

Put all vegetables into slow cooker.
Rub meat with garlic, pepper and paprika.
Place on top of vegetables.
Pour on liquid ingredients.
Place bay leaf on top.

108

v.combat-fat.com www.combat-fat.com www.combat-fat.com www.combat-fat.com www.combat-fat.

Cook on low about 8 hours.
MAKES 8 SERVINGS

RICE PILAF

1 tbsp olive oil
1/2 cup chopped scallion
1/2 cup long grain rice
1/2 cup chopped red pepper
1 cup hot water
1/4 cup dry wine
3 tsp vinegar, divided
1 1/4 tsp Mrs. Dash Lemon Pepper blend, divided
1/2 cup frozen peas
1 diced zucchini

Heat oil in skillet.
Add rice onion and pepper
Cook until rice is golden, stirring constantly.
Gradually stir in water, wine, 2-tsp vinegar and 1 tsp Mrs. Dash.
Bring to boil, reduce heat.
Add vegetables and simmer covered.
Cook until rice and vegetables are tender.
Sprinkle with remaining ingredients, fluff with fork and serve.
MAKES 6 SERVINGS

ROASTED CARROTS WITH LIME

1 1/2 pound carrots
2 tbsp fresh lime juice
2 tbsp water
6 tbsp brown sugar
2 tsp Mrs. Dash Garlic & Herb Blend
Non-stick spray
lime wedges

Peel carrots and cut into thin diagonal slices
Preheat oven to 375 degrees.
Coat 3x9 baking dish with non-stick spray.
Place carrots in a single layer in dish.
Add lime juice and water.
Mix sugar and Mrs. Dash well then drizzle on carrots.
Bake covered 20 minutes.
Turn to coat all sides.
Bake another 5 to 10 minutes uncovered until soft, glazed shiny and slightly brown.
Serve with lime wedges.
MAKES 8 SERVINGS

109

Your New Friend—The Sweet Potato

Ah, the sweet potato! Delicious, wholesome, nutritious. Simple and quick to make in the microwave, or steamed on top of the stove, it can become a regular feature in your dinner menu.

The sweet potato blends with herbs, spices and flavorings producing delicious dishes of all types. From casseroles, salads, breads and desserts, sweet potatoes add valuable, appetizing nutrients and color to any meal.

As a main dish or prepared as a dessert, the sweet potato is a nutritious and economical food. One baked sweet potato (3 1/2 ounce serving) provides over 8,800 IU of vitamin A or about twice the recommended daily allowance, yet it contains only 141 calories making it valuable for the weight watcher. This nutritious vegetable provides 42 percent of the Recommended Daily Allowance (RDA) for vitamin C, 6 percent of the RDA for calcium, 10 percent of the RDA for iron, and 8 percent of the RDA for thiamin for healthy adults. It is low in sodium and is a good source of fiber and other important vitamins and minerals. A complex carbohydrate food source, it provides beta-carotene which may be a factor in reducing the risk of certain cancers.

When buying sweet potatoes, select sound, firm roots. Handle them carefully to prevent bruising. Storage in a dry, unrefrigerated bin kept at 55-60 degrees F. is best. DO NOT REFRIGERATE, because temperatures below 55 degrees F. will chill this tropical vegetable giving it a hard core and an undesirable taste when cooked.

Most sweet potato dishes freeze well. Save time and energy by making a sweet potato dish to serve and one to store in the freezer!

SLOPPY JOES

1 cup boiling water
1 tbsp bottled chili sauce
1 cup dry textured soy protein
1 cup chopped onion
1/2 cup finely chopped zucchini
1/2 cup chopped bell pepper
8 ounce can tomato sauce
1/4 cup bottled chili sauce
1/2 tsp chili powder
2 tsp Worcestershire sauce
1 tsp vinegar
6 hamburger buns

Combine the water and 1 tbsp chili sauce.
Pour over soy protein to rehydrate it.
Sauté the vegetables in a small amount of water until tender.
Add the soy protein mixture, and remaining ingredients.
Simmer 5 minutes.
Serve on hamburger buns.
MAKES 6 SERVINGS

SMASHED POTATOES

4 Yukon gold potatoes cut into cubes
1 tsp butter
1/2 cup liquid nonfat, nondairy creamer
1 tbsp pepper
1 tbsp parsley flakes

Place potatoes in a large pot.
Fill with water 3/4 to top.
Bring to boil.
Reduce heat and simmer for 20 minutes.
Drain and return to pot.
Add butter.
Warm creamer in microwave and add to pot.
Add spices and stir well.
Smash with potato masher and serve.
MAKES 4 SERVINGS

SOUTHWESTERN PORK TENDERLOIN

1 1/2 pounds of pork tenderloin, sliced in half lengthwise
2 tbsp chili powder
1 1/2 tsp oregano

111

3/4 tsp cumin
2 tbsp minced garlic
1 tbsp vegetable oil

Mix all ingredients except pork in a small bowl.
Rub mixture over entire tenderloin.
Cover pork and refrigerate at least 2 hours.
Preheat grill.
Grill for 15 minutes (or until thermometer inserted in the middle reads 160 degrees).
MAKES 6 SERVINGS

SPAGHETTI SQUASH POMODRO

1 spaghetti squash, about 3 pounds
1 tbsp olive oil
2 cups ripe tomatoes
1/2 cup grated Romano cheese
1 tbsp Mrs. Dash Classic Italiano Blend
1/4 cup toasted almonds

Preheat oven to 350 degrees.
Pierce whole squash in 3 places with a knife.
Bake until squash can be easily depressed with a finger.
Cut in half immediately and cool 10 minutes.
Meanwhile, combine remaining ingredients, except nuts, and mix well in large bowl.
Scoop out squash seeds and discard.
Comb strands out of squash with fork until only the shell remains.
Add strands to sauce bowl and mix well.
Top with nuts and serve.
MAKES 4 SERVINGS

SPINACH SALAD

1 pound cleaned, drained raw spinach
1 tbsp olive oil
1/2 cup bacon bits
1/2 cup chopped red onion
1/2 cup vinegar
1 tsp sugar
1/4 tsp dried mustard
1/4 tsp black pepper

Combine spinach with olive oil in large bowl.
Toss well.
Combine remaining ingredients in a small bowl.
Mix well.

112

Pour dressing over spinach and toss.
MAKES 4 SERVINGS

SPUNKY CHILI

2 cans red kidney beans, rinsed and drained
2 cans chunky, chili style tomatoes undrained
1 cup chopped onion
1 cup chopped green bell pepper
1 1/2 tbsp Mrs. Dash Classic Italiano Blend
1 tbsp chili powder
1/2 cup lowfat shredded cheddar cheese

Combine all ingredients except cheddar cheese in large pot.
Simmer covered stirring occasionally for 20 minutes.
Garnish with cheese after serving.
MAKES 6 SERVINGS

Your New Friend — Mrs. Dash

Mrs. Dash is one of those wonderful condiments to have on your shelf. A magical blend of herbs and spices, completely fat-free yet flavor rich, it boasts an additional health benefit for all—no salt added!

My mother first introduced me to Mrs. Dash years ago. She uses it in everything from soups to stews, salads to pasta dishes.

Tossed on a chicken breast which is then cooked in the microwave or on your counter top grill—voila! you've got a tasty dish for lunch or supper.

Mrs. Dash comes in a variety of unique blends and can be found on your grocer's shelves.

113

STRAWBERRY ORANGE MUFFINS

1 cup chopped strawberries
1/3 cup sugar
1 tbsp orange juice
1 1/2 cups whole wheat flour
1/2 cup soy flour
2 tsp baking powder
1 tsp baking soda
1/2 tsp nutmeg
2/3 cup orange juice
2 tbsp canola oil
2 lightly beaten egg whites
1 1/2 tsp freshly grated orange peel

Preheat oven to 350 degrees.
Mix strawberries, sugar and 1 tbsp orange juice.
Set aside.
Combine flours, baking powder and baking soda in a large mixing bowl.
Combine orange juice, oil and egg whites in smaller bowl.
Whisk well.
Add liquid ingredients to dry ingredients.
Mix until blended.
Stir in strawberry mixture and orange peel.
Pour into non-stick muffin cups.
Bake for 15 minutes.
MAKES 12 MUFFINS

STRAWBERRY SYRUP

1/2 cup pancake syrup
1/2 cup sliced strawberries (if frozen, thaw prior to cooking)

Combine syrup and berries in microwave safe dish
Cover with plastic wrap
Microwave until mixture begins to boil
Let stand for 1 minute and serve

STOVETOP LENTIL CASSEROLE

2 cans lentil soup
1 finely diced carrot
2 tsp Mrs. Dash Classic Italiano Blend
1 cup chunky tomato sauce
3 ounces Healthy Choice Smoked Sausage
2 chopped scallions

Combine all but last 3 ingredients in a pot.

114

Bring to boil, stirring often.
Reduce heat and simmer 5 minutes
Mash lentils with potato masher until half appear mashed.
Add tomato sauce and sausage.
Simmer 10 more minutes.
Garnish with onions.
MAKES 6 SERVINGS

TERIYAKI STEAK FINGERS

2 pounds sirloin steak, trimmed of fat
1/2 cup light soy sauce
1/4 cup vinegar
2 tbsp brown sugar
2 tbsp-minced onions
1 tbsp canola oil
1 tbsp-minced garlic
1/2 tsp ground ginger
1/4 tsp pepper
8 wooden skewers.

Soak skewers in water.
Cut steak into 1/2 inch strips.
Put steak into a large bowl.
Add remaining ingredients to bowl and mix well.
Cover and refrigerate at least 2 hours.
Thread meat strips onto skewers.
Grill to desired doneness (3 to 5 minutes).
MAKES 8 SERVINGS.

THAI PASTA SALAD

3/4 cup water
2 tbsp vinegar
2 tbsp lite soy sauce
1/4cup peanut butter
2 tbsp sugar
1/4 tsp cayenne pepper
1 clove garlic, minced
2 tsp ginger
1/2 pkg silken tofu
1 cup fresh green soybeans
1/2 pound snowpeas, cut in 1 inch pieces
1 chopped red pepper
1 cup broccoli florets
2 thinly sliced carrots
8 ounces vermicelli, broken in half

115

1 tsp sesame oil
1/4 cup chopped scallions

Combine first 9 ingredients in blender.
Puree.
Refrigerate, this is the dressing.

Put soybeans in pot, cover with water.
Simmer until tender, about 15 minutes.
Blanch the remaining vegetables except onion, in boiling water for 1 minute.
Drain.
Cook vermicelli according to package.
Rinse with cold water and toss with soybeans and vegetables.
Refrigerate at least 2 hours.
Toss with dressing prior to serving.
Garnish with onions.
MAKES 10 SERVINGS

Your New Friend — Garlic

Chopped, crushed, powdered, flaked, whole—you name it, it's available and adds some great flavor to your meals. Bought in bulk at a buyer's club, like Costco or B.J.'s, it is very affordable and keeps for a long time in the kitchen. Add it to sauces, salad dressings, and marinades, eat it straight if you want.

Medical studies have shown that garlic can lower cholesterol, prevent dangerous blood clots, reduce blood pressure, prevent cancer, and protect against bacterial and fungal infections.

In fact, garlic has been used medicinally for at least 3,000 years, but until relatively recently its benefits were considered little more than folklore. According to a report in the *Journal of the American Medical Association* the therapeutic roles of garlic have been described in more than 1,000 scientific studies!

116

VEGGIE PITA SANDWICH

1/8 cup alp alpha sprouts
2 slices tomato, chopped
1/4 cucumber thinly sliced
1/8 cup shredded carrots
2 tbsp black olive slices
1/4 cup plain yogurt
1 tsp lemon juice
2 tbsp lowfat Italian salad dressing
1/4 cup shredded red cabbage
1 whole wheat pita cut into two pockets

Mix yogurt, lemon juice and salad dressing in bowl
Stir in all veggies
Stuff into pita pockets
MAKES 2 SERVINGS

VEGGIE PIZZA

12 inch thick pizza crust
5 ounces pizza sauce
4 ounces lowfat, grated mozzarella cheese
1/4 cup grated Parmesan cheese
1/2 cup chopped mushrooms
1/2 cup sliced bell pepper
1/2 cup chopped fresh broccoli
1/2 cup chopped scallions

Preheat oven to 450 degrees.
Place pizza crust on cookie sheet.
Spread pizza sauce on crust
Sprinkle on vegetables.
Top with cheese.
Bake for 7 to 9 minutes.
Cool a few minutes.
Cut and serve.
MAKES 8 SERVINGS

WALDORF SALAD

1 tbsp lemon juice
1 tbsp orange juice
1-tsp sugar
2 tbsp nonfat milk
1/3 cup lowfat mayonnaise
2 apples (any variety) cored and cut into cubes

117

3 celery stalks, chopped
1/2 cup raisins
1/2 cup walnuts

In large bowl combine the first 5 ingredients.
Mix well.
Add remaining ingredients and toss.
MAKES 2 SERVINGS

WHOLE WHEAT PANCAKES

1 cup whole wheat flour
1/2 tsp baking soda
1/2 tsp baking powder
11/2 tsp granulated sugar
1/4 cup egg substitute
1 cup nonfat milk
1 tbsp canola oil
1/4 tsp vanilla

Combine dry ingredients in a large bowl
Combine wet ingredients in a small bowl and whisk well
Coat skillet with non-stick spray
Over high heat, pour in batter for 4 pancakes
After mixture stops bubbling, turn
Cook another minute or so until done
MAKES 8 SERVINGS

6
Combat Fat!
Menus

The following pages provide a sample 8-week menu for you to follow. Of course, everyone has his or her own likes and dislikes, so feel free to substitute from the appropriate catagories as needed.

You'll also find blank menus in the back of the book so you can build your own. Whichever way you go, the key concept is to stick to an intelligent eating plan. Avoid excess snacking. Avoid foods that are not listed as "acceptable". Stick with your portion control!

Achieving a healthy fat percentage to weight ratio comes down to comes down to calorie management. If you intake more calories than you expend, you will put on fat. If you intake fewer calories than you expend, you will lose fat. Wise calorie management is at the heart of a smart eating plan.

Combat Fat! strives to encourage you to eat wisely by giving you the knowledge and guidelines to make good nutritional decisions for you and your family.

The supermarkets are filled will everything you need to follow the Combat Fat! plan. There is no need to buy expensive supplements or foods. Simple, healthy, delicious nutrition is just a matter of choice and habit. So…make good food choices and follow healthy eating habits!

Combat Fat! Sample Menu Week 1

	BREAKFAST	LUNCH	DINNER	SNACK
MONDAY	2	7	18	10
TUESDAY	8	4	17	25
WEDNESDAY	3	8	24	9
THURSDAY	13	6	14	5
FRIDAY	9	17	25	7
SATURDAY	12	15	4	20
SUNDAY	5	7	9	12

Combat Fat! Sample Menu Week 2

	BREAKFAST	LUNCH	DINNER	SNACK
MONDAY	10	2	8	2
TUESDAY	6	17	1	23
WEDNESDAY	7	5	21	13
THURSDAY	4	16	13	1
FRIDAY	11	18	11	14
SATURDAY	5	9	2	16
SUNDAY	3	14	19	4

Combat Fat! Sample Menu Week 3

	BREAKFAST	LUNCH	DINNER	SNACK
MONDAY	10	13	5	15
TUESDAY	9	11	10	11
WEDNESDAY	2	10	6	21
THURSDAY	12	12	16	6
FRIDAY	13	21	23	27
SATURDAY	1	19	15	19
SUNDAY	6	22	3	17

Combat Fat! Sample Menu Week 4

	BREAKFAST	LUNCH	DINNER	SNACK
MONDAY	11	20	22	8
TUESDAY	7	17	20	3
WEDNESDAY	8	2	4	24
THURSDAY	4	23	23	23
FRIDAY	23	18	11	18
SATURDAY	12	22	18	26
SUNDAY	7	12	13	2

123

Combat Fat! Sample Menu Week 5

	BREAKFAST	LUNCH	DINNER	SNACK
MONDAY	4	19	2	3
TUESDAY	2	4	10	5
WEDNESDAY	9	3	16	12
THURSDAY	8	5	14	20
FRIDAY	5	21	15	16
SATURDAY	10	9	3	17
SUNDAY	6	15	8	25

124

Combat Fat! Sample Menu Week 6

	BREAKFAST	LUNCH	DINNER	SNACK
MONDAY	13	8	24	1
TUESDAY	11	7	21	7
WEDNESDAY	1	10	6	12
THURSDAY	3	14	19	18
FRIDAY	9	18	11	24
SATURDAY	7	2	17	11
SUNDAY	13	9	1	6

Combat Fat! Sample Menu Week 7

	BREAKFAST	LUNCH	DINNER	SNACK
MONDAY	8	18	11	24
TUESDAY	7	2	17	11
WEDNESDAY	13	9	1	6
THURSDAY	8	17	7	19
FRIDAY	12	13	12	15
SATURDAY	11	20	23	22
SUNDAY	3	1	20	23

Combat Fat! Sample Menu Week 8

	BREAKFAST	LUNCH	DINNER	SNACK
MONDAY	2	6	25	9
TUESDAY	5	11	5	23
WEDNESDAY	4	3	22	27
THURSDAY	10	21	19	10
FRIDAY	1	2	3	14
SATURDAY	2	12	18	4
SUNDAY	5	6	7	13

127

7
Combat Fat!
Workouts

There is no better feeling than to feel fit and strong. You'll look better, have more energy, possess more confidence, and you'll have a more positive outlook on life!

In this section, you will find an exercise program that will suit you—whatever your fitness level. Even if you haven't exercised in years, you can start today by following our EZ Basic Workout plan. If you want to take it up a notch, our Advanced Workout is just what you'll need. If you are an experienced and regular exerciser and are seeking a workout plan that includes precision body sculpting, look no further! The Elite Workout will give you the body you've always dreamed of.

Of course, with any exercise program, whether you a starting anew or increasing the intensity of your workouts, you should consult your doctor and receive his or her permission.

Remember that Rome was not built in a day—so don't expect to see changes overnight. It takes time to gain the results from regular exercise…but the rewards are well worth it. Recognize, too, that "the first is the worst": the first day, the first week, the first month will be your toughest.

Stay with it. One morning you'll look in the mirror and see a new you!

Exercise 101

Along with eating properly and monitoring your body fat levels, exercise is a vital component of the Combat Fat! Program. The Report of the Surgeon General in 1996 made it crystal clear: America has got to get moving; if only for 30 minutes each day! Of course, it's even better if you can do more. We have developed three levels of extensive 8-week workouts (basic, advanced and elite) for you to follow, or to use as a guide, as you successfully change your lifestyle for the better. Once you complete each 8-week cycle, you can move to the next level. But before plunging into the workouts, let's review some of the basics about exercise.

What Type of Exercise Should I Do?

There are five major components to fitness: cardiovascular fitness, muscular strength and endurance, flexibility, and body composition. In order to be fit, you need to make sure that you cover all these areas in your workouts. In other words, your workout program should include cardiovascular training, flexibility exercises, and strength training. If you do one without the other two, you shortchange yourself in terms of benefits and may leave yourself more susceptible to injury.

Cardiovascular Training

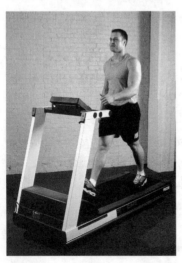

Cardiovascular training is exercise that increases the efficiency and health of your heart and lungs, and includes large-range of motion activities such as running, jogging, stair climbing, fast walking and biking. There are two types of cardio training: aerobic and anaerobic. In aerobic exercise your body uses oxygen; this type of training involves moving large muscle groups, such as your legs, for a sustained period of time (at least 20 minutes). Examples of aerobic exercise include fast walking, jogging and biking. Anaerobic exercise does not use

130

WHAT IS MY TARGET HEART RATE?

Your target heart rate is really a range that estimates how hard you are working out. The low and high ends of your target heart rate range are estimated by the following formula: (220-your age) multiplied by .60 and .85. For example, if you are 20 years old your estimated target heart rate range would be as follows:

$$220-20=200$$
$$200 * .60 = 120$$
$$200 * .85 = 170$$

Your target heart rate range would be 120 – 170 beats per minute.

While this formula only provides a general estimate, it can be a helpful tool in gauging how hard you are working. To follow the Surgeon General's recommendation that you do at least 30 minutes of moderate activity every day, you should try to get your heart rate up to at least the low end of your range for 30 minutes. You can calculate your heart rate by taking your pulse at your wrist for 10 seconds and then multiplying by 6 to get your beats per minute. Or, you can purchase a heart-rate monitor, which digitally displays your heart rate on a watch.

Another important thing to consider is your recovery heart rate. This is your heart rate, in beats per minutes, after resting for one minute following your cardiovascular activity. Your heart rate should drop at least 20 beats one minute after you stop exercising. The more fit you are, the faster and more your heart rate will drop. If you find that your heart rate is not dropping, you should lower the intensity of your exercise until you become more fit. In general when doing cardiovascular aerobic exercise you should feel like you are working moderately hard to hard, but should never be working out so hard that you cannot talk or are severely short of breath.

oxygen, and is associated with higher intensity short bursts of energy (such as jumping or sprinting). Both aerobic and anaerobic cardiovascular exercise burn calories and therefore each is useful. However, while aerobic exercise tends to burn fat in your body, anaerobic exercise burns glycogen (stored carbohydrates). Therefore, to focus on burning fat, we recommend you do aerobic exercise in your target heart rate range for at least 20 minutes.

Flexibility Training

Flexibility is the range of motion that you have at your joints. While exercisers and non-exercisers alike often neglect it, it is extremely important to stretch your muscles in order to increase that range of motion and prevent injury. You should stretch both before and after your exercise or activity. Before you exercise, your warm-up stretch should involve doing a less intense version of whatever your main activity will be. For example, if you are going for a two-mile jog, your warm-up stretch would be a five to ten minute walk. After your activity, you should do static stretching, which is when you hold a stretch position for 15-20 seconds. In addition, it is a good idea to do stretches in the morning and before you go to sleep at night. You will find a great static stretch program for all the major muscles in this chapter.

Strength Training

Strength training helps to build lean mass—exactly what we want to Combat Fat! You can do strength training with dumbbells, exercise machines, soup cans, even your own body weight. The key is to load your body with resistance against gravity. Several studies have shown that people who have more muscle, or lean body mass, actually burn more calories at rest than people who are not muscular. The reason for this is that muscles require more energy than fat. By incorporating strength training into your exercise program you will elevate your resting metabolism, reduce your percentage of body fat, and look more toned and defined. Strength training also is the most important thing you can do to offset the gravitational effects of aging. (After age 30 we can lose up to a half-pound of lean body

132

mass each year if we don't do strength training). In addition, strength training helps protect you from injury, and is vital for the prevention of osteoporosis—a degenerative disease of the bones that occurs quite commonly in women—because weight bearing exercise has been shown to actually increase bone density.

When you do strength training, there are several things you should bear in mind: first, make sure that you do not use weight that is too heavy or too light. A good rule of thumb is to use a weight that enables you to do about eight to ten repetitions (repeated movements of an exercise) in good form before you begin to get fatigued in the muscle. Second, it is essential to use a strong, controlled contraction of the muscles you are working, rather than momentum when performing each exercise. And, third watch yourself in a mirror to make sure you are lifting weights with proper form (knees slightly bend, no arching your back or leaning forward or back).

How Often Should I Exercise?

The Combat Fat! Workout programs that you will find at the end of this chapter fall into three categories, depending upon your current fitness level. We provide a progressive eight-week program that includes both cardiovascular and weight training guidelines. (Also, remember to stretch every day). Our program is designed on an optimal five-day per week workout schedule, and each workout ranges from 30minutes to over an hour in duration. However, you can also realize gains working out three days a week, but of course it will take longer and the process will be slower. Even if you can't get your "official" workout in make sure that you are PHYSICALLY ACTIVE each and every day of the week. By physically active we mean walk to the store instead of driving the car, do some gardening, climb the stairs instead of using the elevator. If you just think a little creatively you will see that there are countless opportunities to fit activity into your daily life and to make it become as routine as getting dressed in the morning. The more active you are, the more calories you burn, the less fat you lug around. It's as simple as that.

133

The Combat Fat! Workout At-A-Glance

It has never been easier to follow a comprehensive and effective exercise program than before. We have endeavored to make the Combat Fat! workout simple to follow and geared to your needs.

EZ Basic—This is for individuals who have not exercised in years and are just beginning a fitness program. We will ease you into your program. You need no equipment except for a pair of comfortable shoes, an exercise mat, and two light dumbbells or soup cans. **Go to page 151.**

Advanced—This program is designed for men and women who are reasonably fit. While a gym membership is not essential, you will need access to dumbbells. **Go to page 169.**

Elite—An intensive, body-sculpting program for those who seek a challenge. This program requires the kind of equipment found in most health clubs or gyms. **Go to page 192.**

Each workout program consists of stretching, strength training, and cardiovascular segments. The stretches for all the workouts are the same and begin on the following page.

Reps and Sets—On the workout charts, the word **reps** refers to the number of times you repeat a particular exercise. The word **set** refers to a number of repetitions performed without rest. So, if you were to do 2 sets of 10 reps for squats, you would perform 10 squats, rest for about 15-20 seconds, then perform another 10 squats. Perform each rep slowly with control. Always breathe out during the exertion phase of the exercise. To increase the difficulty or intensity of your workouts over time you can use heavier resistance (more weight) or increase the number of sets and reps.

Your goal is to fatigue the muscles you are working by the end of a set.

134

.combat-fat.com www.combat-fat.com www.combat-fat.com www.combat-fat.com www.combat-fat.

STRETCHES

Stretching is important for a number of reasons:

- It relieves tension, which leads to head, back and neck aches.

- It prevents injuries by increasing the range of motion in your joints.

- It prepares the body for exercising by warming muscles and increasing the blood flow throughout the body.

Before you start any workout program, no matter how easy it appears, you should stretch daily for a full week to build flexibility. This is especially true if you have not exercised in a long time. Being flexible means you can move your body freely and without pain through a full range of motion.

If you have not exercised in several years, you should perform every stretch in this book for a full week—before attempting any of the exercises!

A good stretch is one that is slow and easy with no bouncing motion. You should hold each stretch for about 15 to 20 seconds and repeat the stretch two to three times. You should never push a stretch to the point of pain. If you feel pain, relax! This is your body's way of indicating that something is wrong. It is recommended that you stretch every night before you go to sleep. **For better results, you should stretch in the morning and evening.**

Also remember to do an active warm-up prior to exercising (jumping jacks, fast walking) and repeat the stretching routine after your workout.

135

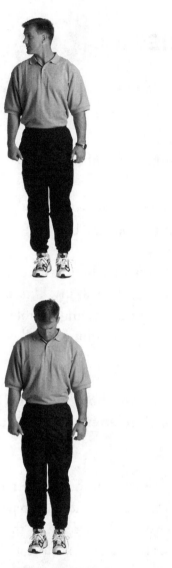
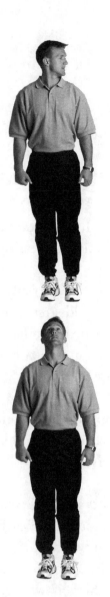

Neck Stretches

Look to the left, right, up, and down, by turning your head slowly in these directions as shown. Your neck should move as if you were nodding "yes" and "no." Hold each motion for 15 seconds. Be careful! You do not want to raise, lower, or rotate your neck too much. You can cause severe neck injury this way, so be sure to always use slow and relaxing motions.

136

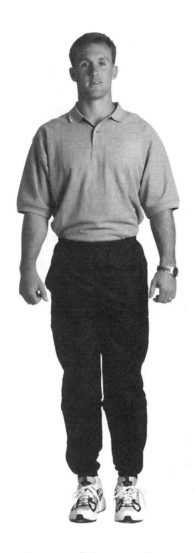
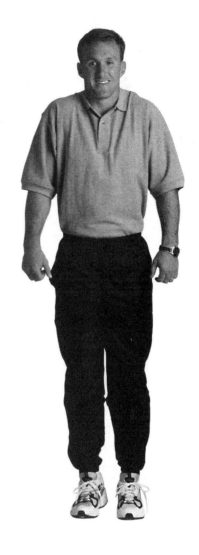

Shoulder Stretch

Rotate your shoulders slowly up and down, keeping your arms relaxed at your sides. This stretch will help relieve the pressure on the base of your neck, keeping this area from tightening and causing pain and headaches.

You will begin your stretching routine with neck and shoulder stretches every day, but you can also use these stretches throughout the day as tension builds. You can actually relieve or prevent headaches by simply keeping your neck and shoulders loose.

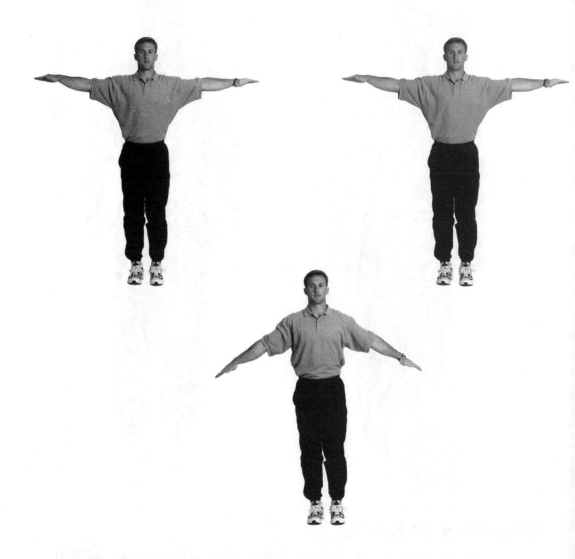

Arm Circles

From a standing or sitting position, rotate your arms slowly in big circles. This will loosen your shoulders and prepare them for exercises such as pushups, dips, and arm kickbacks. Arm circles are also good stress relievers, because they help relax the shoulder muscles that are connected to the base of your neck.

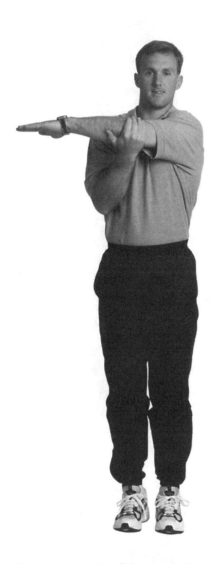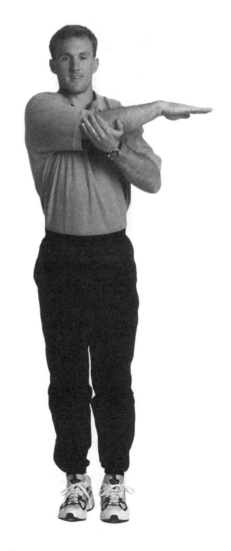

Arm and Shoulder Stretch

Pull your right arm across your chest with your left hand placed on your right elbow as shown. Hold for 10 seconds, and then repeat with the other arm.

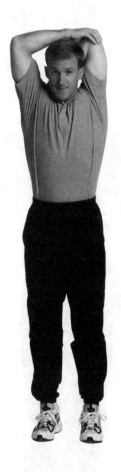
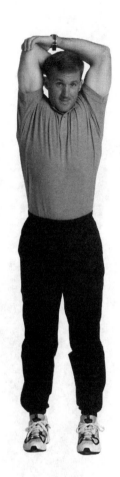

Triceps Stretch

Put both arms over and behind your head as shown. Grab your right elbow with your left hand and pull your elbow toward your opposite shoulder. Lean with the pull. Repeat with the other arm. You should hold this stretch for 15 seconds.

This stretch will help to stretch the triceps muscle, located in the back of the upper arm. You will firm this area by performing various types of pushups, dips, and isolation exercises.

140

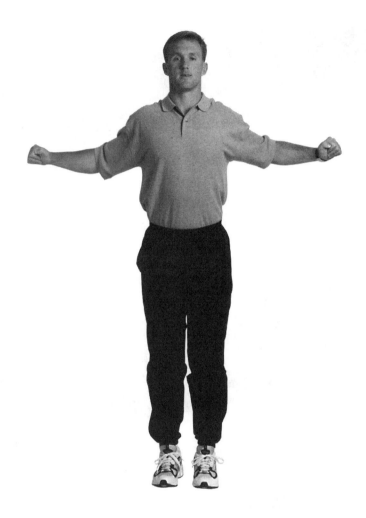

Chest Stretch

Stand with your upper arms parallel to the floor as shown. Slowly pull your elbows back slowly as far as you can. Hold for 15 seconds.

This chest stretch aids in preparing the chest and shoulder muscles for pushups and dips. Having flexibility in the upper torso will also help to prevent injury.

141

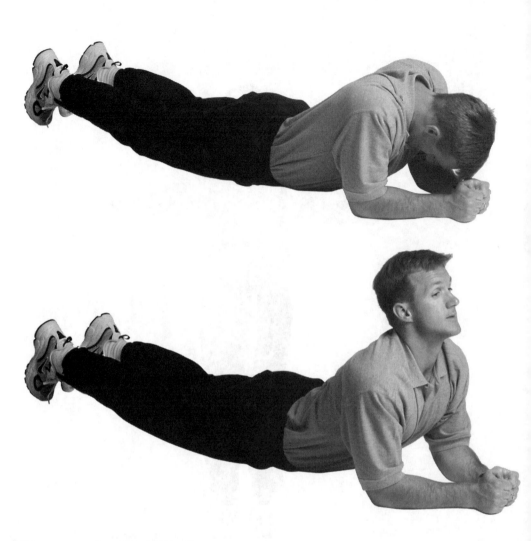

Stomach Stretch

Lay on your stomach. Push yourself up on your elbows and leave your abdomen and legs flat on the ground. Slowly and carefully raise your head and shoulders. Be careful not to arch your back too much. Hold for 15 seconds and then repeat.

Before you perform any crunches, you need to thoroughly stretch your stomach muscles. This will help you achieve a full range of motion for any ab exercises.

142

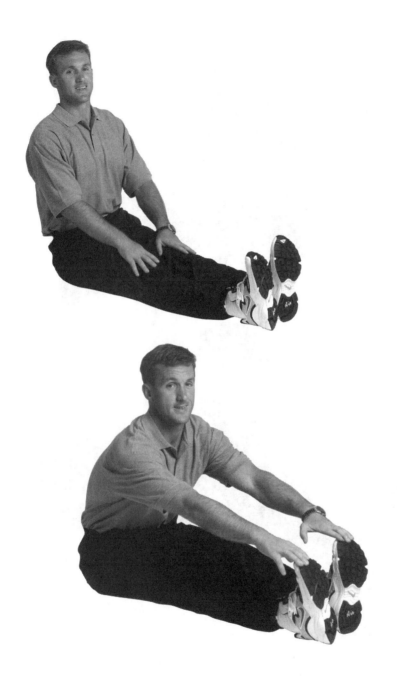

Toe Touch

Sit on the floor with your legs in front of you. Lean toward your toes and grab your ankles. Hold for 15 seconds. Do not lock your knees!

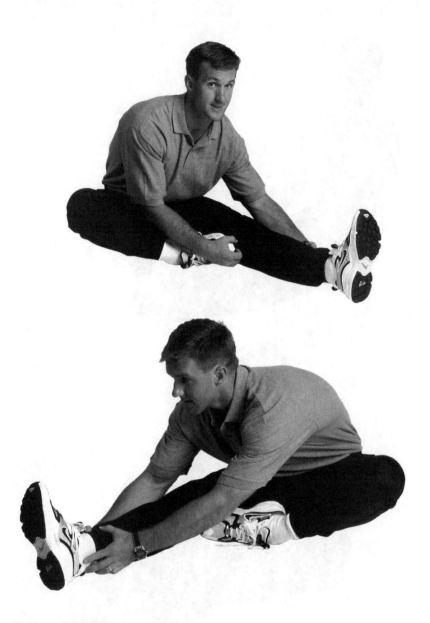

Hurdler Stride

Sit on the floor with your legs straight in front of you. Bend your right knee and place the bottom of your foot on the inside of your opposite thigh. With your back straight, lean forward in order to stretch the back of your legs (hamstrings) and your lower back. Hold the stretch for 15 seconds.

144

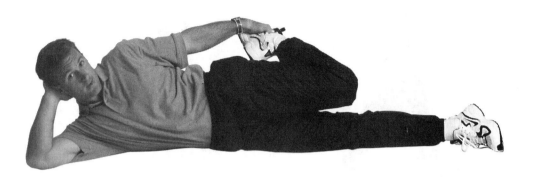

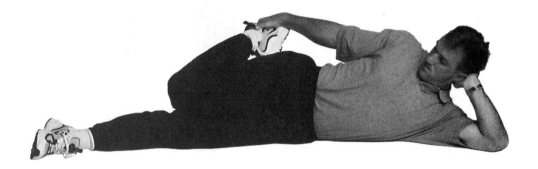

Thigh Stretch

Lay on your right side. Grab your left foot with your left hand and slowly pull your foot toward your buttocks. Hold the stretch for 15 seconds, and then switch sides. You can also perform this stretch standing.

It is important to keep your knees as close together as possible during this stretch. When performing leg exercises, you will need flexibility in your upper thigh area to reach a full range of motion and receive maximum benefits.

145

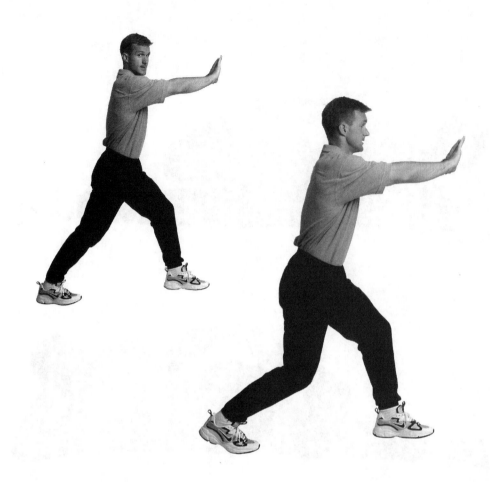

Calf Stretch

Stand with one foot approximately two to three feet in front of your other foot in the stride position as shown. Bend your front leg forward, keeping your rear leg straight. Lean forward until you feel your rear calf muscle stretch. Make sure your toes are pointing in the direction you are facing. Hold for 15 seconds and repeat with the other leg.

As a modification of this exercise, and to stretch your Achilles tendon, simply bend your rear knee while in the same position as shown. This modification will completely stretch the lower leg and aid in preventing tendonitis in that area.

146

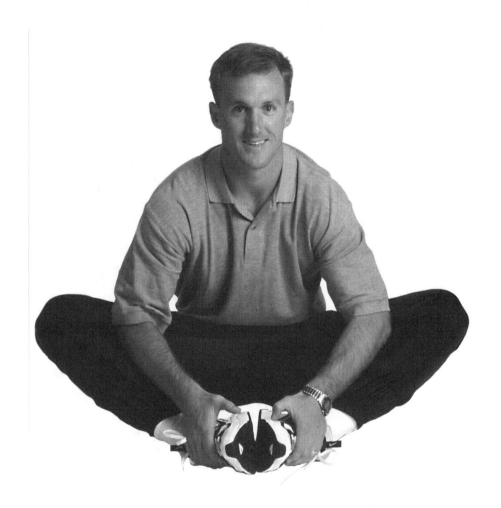

Butterfly Stretch

Sit on your buttocks, with your legs bent and the soles of your feet together. Grab your ankles and place your elbows on your inner thighs. Slowly push down with your elbows.

This stretch helps to tone and loosen the inner thigh region.

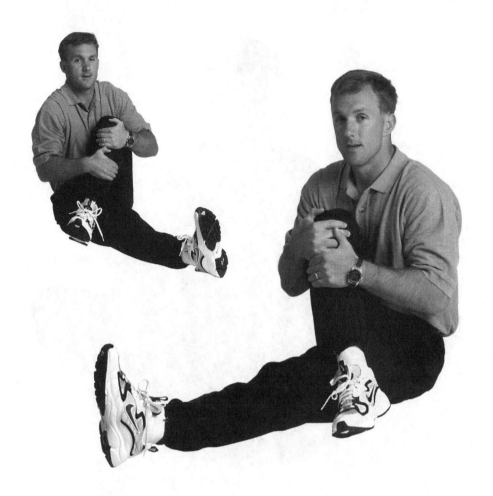

Hip/Buttocks Stretch

Sit on the ground with your legs crossed in front of you. Keeping your legs crossed, bring your right leg up so that your foot is placed flat on the ground next to your left knee. Pull your right leg all the way to your chest and hold for 15 seconds. Repeat with the other leg.

Before and after walking, running, or performing any lower body calisthenics exercises, make sure to properly stretch this tendon. This will prevent what is commonly known as "overuse injuries" in the hip and the knee. Keeping this area flexible is crucial to any fitness program.

148

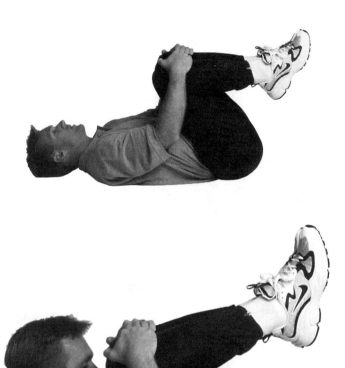

Lower Back Stretch

Lay flat on your back. Pull your knees to your stomach region and hold with both arms as shown for 20 seconds.

As you may know, the lower back is probably the most commonly injured area of the body. Many lower back strains are caused by inactivity, lack of flexibility, and overuse, such as lifting heavy objects improperly.

149

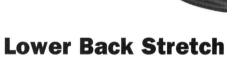

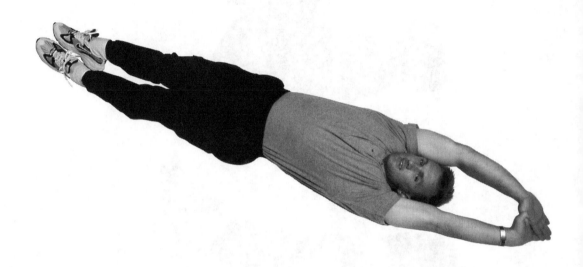

Full Body Stretch

Lay flat on the floor with your arms extended over your head and your lower back flat on the floor but not arched. Slowly stretch your entire body—try to make yourself an inch taller!

This is another great tension reliever after a tough day.

Combat Fat!

EZ BASIC WORKOUT

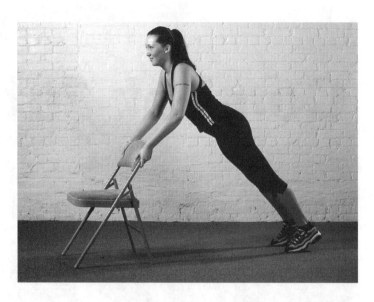

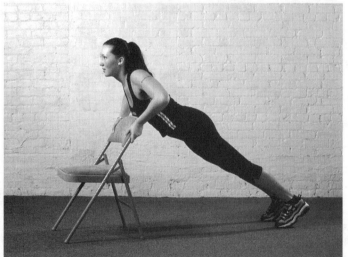

Chair Push-up

Lean against a sturdy chair or table with your feet together and push away from the chair as you would from the ground in a regular push-up. You'll be working your chest muscles and building your strength to do regular push-ups.

152

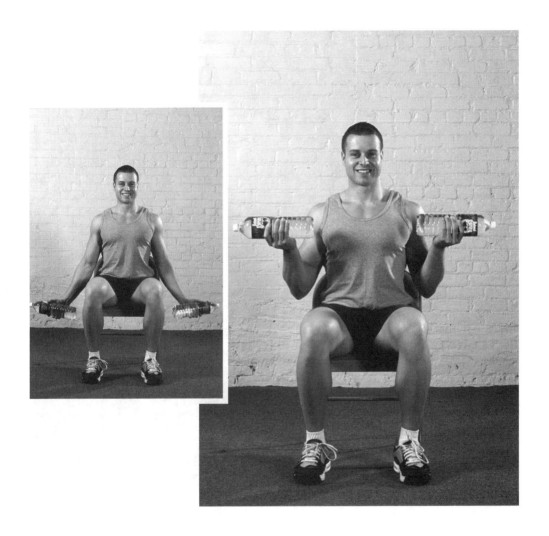

Seated Biceps Curls

Keep your elbows next to your sides and your back straight. Lift your hands to your chest by bending your arms at the elbows. Repeat.

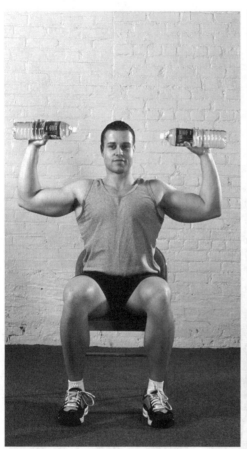 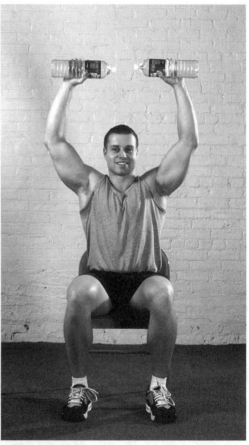

Seated Shoulder Press

Sit straight in a chair with a weight in each hand. Exhale as you push the weights over your head until your arms are almost fully extended. Slowly lower them to shoulder height and repeat.

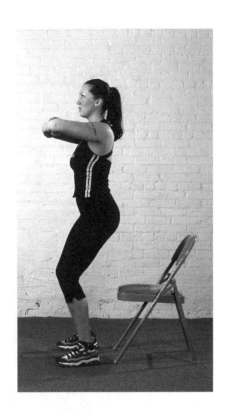 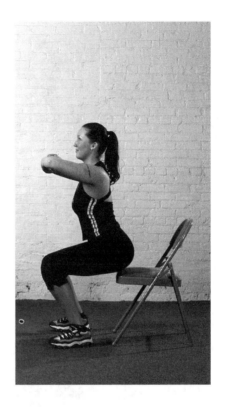

Chair Squat

Stand in front of a chair, sit down and repeat the process of standing and sitting. Keep your back straight, your head up, and your feet about shoulder width apart. Do not bend your knees beyond a 90 degree angle. Perform this exercise with your feet flat on the floor at all times. This exercise is excellent for toning your legs and buttocks.

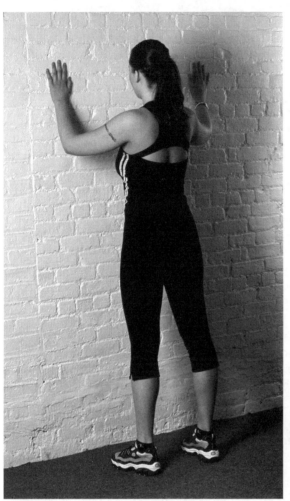 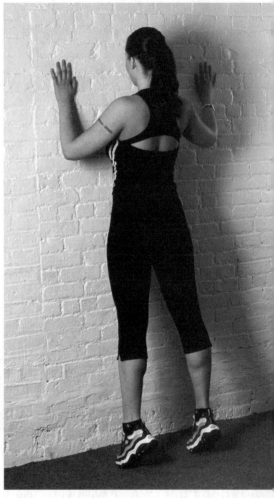

Heel Raise

Lean slightly against a wall. Lift yourself up onto your toes and then lower yourself down slowly. This exercise tones and strengthens your calf muscles.

156

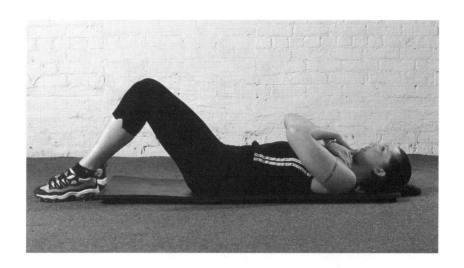

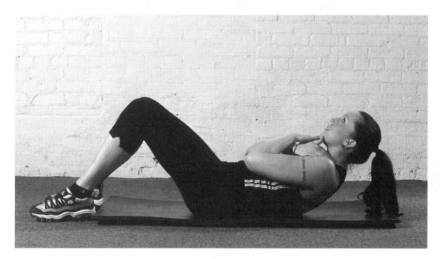

Crunch

Lay on your back as shown. Cross your hands over your chest and bring your shoulders off the floor while contracting your abdominal muscles. Be careful not to lift your torso more than shown as this can be damaging to your lower back.

157

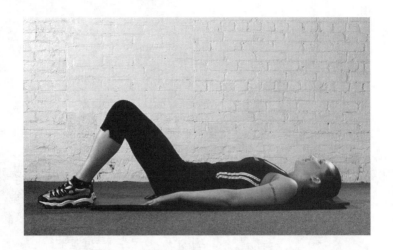

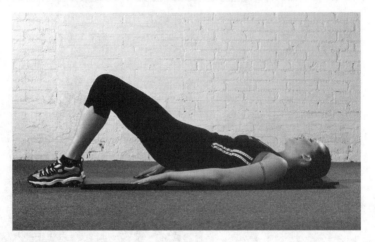

Pelvic Tilt

Lay on your back with your knees bent and your feet and hands on the floor. Flex your buttocks as you lift your hips off the floor. Lower slowly and repeat. Your shoulders should remain flat on the floor throughout the exercise.

For maximum benefit, hold the "up" position for three to five seconds before lowering your hips back to the ground.

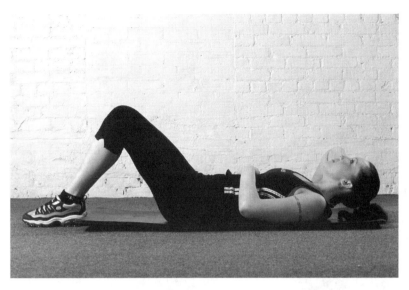

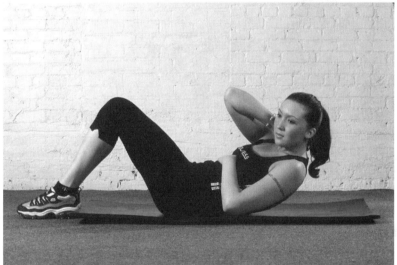

Oblique Crunch

Lay on your back with your knees bent and your feet on the floor. Lift your chest off the floor, twisting to bring your right elbow to your left knee. Switch sides and repeat.

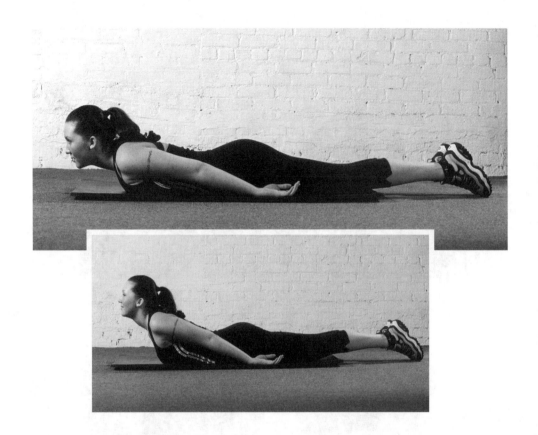

Hyperextension

Lay face down, with your hands resting at the sides of your body. Slowly raise your torso about 2-3 inches from the ground, and hold for a 3-second count. This small movement helps strengthen your lower back. When you begin raising your torso, slightly arch your upper back, shoulders and head. If you encounter any type of pain during this exercise, STOP! Also, do not fatigue your lower back muscles. Stop when you start to feel a tight sensation.

160

Combat Fat! EZ Basic Workout Week #1

DAY #1   DAY #2   DAY #3   DAY #4   DAY #5

FLEXIBILITY

All stretches should be performed daily.

RESISTANCE EXERCISES

Chair Squat	10	10	10	10	10
Chair Push-up	5	5	5	5	5
Crunch	5	5	5	5	5
Seated Bicep Curls					
Pelvic Tilt					
Heel Raise					
Seated Shoulder Press					
Oblique Crunch					
Hyperextension					

CARDIOVASCULAR EXERCISE

Fast Walk	10	10	10	10	10

161

Combat Fat! EZ Basic Workout Week #2

| DAY #1 | DAY #2 | DAY #3 | DAY #4 | DAY #5 |

FLEXIBILITY

All stretches should be performed daily.

RESISTANCE EXERCISES

Chair Squat	10	10	10	10	10
Chair Push-up	5	5	5	5	5
Crunch	5	5	5	5	5
Seated Bicep Curls	8	8	8	8	8
Pelvic Tilt	10	10	10	10	10
Heel Raise	10	10	10	10	10
Seated Shoulder Press					
Oblique Crunch					
Hyperextension					

CARDIOVASCULAR EXERCISE

Fast Walk	12	12	12	12	12

162

Combat Fat! EZ Basic Workout Week #3

DAY #1	DAY #2	DAY #3	DAY #4	DAY #5

FLEXIBILITY

All stretches should be performed daily.

RESISTANCE EXERCISES

Chair Squat	10	10	10	10	10
Chair Push-up	5	5	5	5	5
Crunch	5	5	5	5	5
Seated Bicep Curls	8	8	8	8	8
Pelvic Tilt	10	10	10	10	10
Heel Raise	10	10	10	10	10
Seated Shoulder Press	10	10	10	10	10
Oblique Crunch	5	5	5	5	5
Hyperextension	5	5	5	5	5

CARDIOVASCULAR EXERCISE

Fast Walk	15	15	15	15	15

Combat Fat! EZ Basic Workout Week #4

| DAY #1 | DAY #2 | DAY #3 | DAY #4 | DAY #5 |

FLEXIBILITY

All stretches should be performed daily.

RESISTANCE EXERCISES

Chair Squat	13	13	13	13	13
Chair Push-up	8	8	8	8	8
Crunch	8	8	8	8	8
Seated Bicep Curls	10	10	10	10	10
Pelvic Tilt	12	12	12	12	12
Heel Raise	12	12	12	12	12
Seated Shoulder Press	12	12	12	12	12
Oblique Crunch	8	8	8	8	8
Hyperextension	8	8	8	8	8

CARDIOVASCULAR EXERCISE

Fast Walk	17	17	17	17	17

Combat Fat! EZ Basic Workout Week #5

DAY #1   **DAY #2**   **DAY #3**   **DAY #4**   **DAY #5**

FLEXIBILITY

All stretches should be performed daily.

RESISTANCE EXERCISES

Chair Squat	13	13	13	13	13
Chair Push-up	10	10	10	10	10
Crunch	10	10	10	10	10
Seated Bicep Curls	12	12	12	12	12
Pelvic Tilt	15	15	15	15	15
Heel Raise	15	15	15	15	15
Seated Shoulder Press	15	15	15	15	15
Oblique Crunch	10	10	10	10	10
Hyperextension	10	10	10	10	10

CARDIOVASCULAR EXERCISE

Fast Walk	20	20	20	20	20

Combat Fat! EZ Basic Workout Week #6

DAY #1	DAY #2	DAY #3	DAY #4	DAY #5

FLEXIBILITY

All stretches should be performed daily.

RESISTANCE EXERCISES

	DAY #1	DAY #2	DAY #3	DAY #4	DAY #5
Chair Squat	15	15	15	15	15
Chair Push-up	12	12	12	12	12
Crunch	12	12	12	12	12
Seated Bicep Curls	12	12	12	12	12
Pelvic Tilt	15	15	15	15	15
Heel Raise	15	15	15	15	15
Seated Shoulder Press	15	15	15	15	15
Oblique Crunch	12	12	12	12	12
Hyperextension	12	12	12	12	12

CARDIOVASCULAR EXERCISE

	DAY #1	DAY #2	DAY #3	DAY #4	DAY #5
Fast Walk	22	22	22	22	22

166

Combat Fat! EZ Basic Workout Week #7

DAY #1   DAY #2   DAY #3   DAY #4   DAY #5

FLEXIBILITY

All stretches should be performed daily.

RESISTANCE EXERCISES

	DAY #1	DAY #2	DAY #3	DAY #4	DAY #5
Chair Squat	15	15	15	15	15
Chair Push-up	15	15	15	15	15
Crunch	15	15	15	15	15
Seated Bicep Curls	15	15	15	15	15
Pelvic Tilt	15	15	15	15	15
Heel Raise	15	15	15	15	15
Seated Shoulder Press	15	15	15	15	15
Oblique Crunch	15	15	15	15	15
Hyperextension	15	15	15	15	15

CARDIOVASCULAR EXERCISE

	DAY #1	DAY #2	DAY #3	DAY #4	DAY #5
Fast Walk	25	25	25	25	25

167

Combat Fat! EZ Basic Workout Week #8

DAY #1   **DAY #2**   **DAY #3**   **DAY #4**   **DAY #5**

FLEXIBILITY

All stretches should be performed daily.

RESISTANCE EXERCISES

Chair Squat	15	15	15	15	15
Chair Push-up	15	15	15	15	15
Crunch	15	15	15	15	15
Seated Bicep Curls	15	15	15	15	15
Pelvic Tilt	15	15	15	15	15
Heel Raise	15	15	15	15	15
Seated Shoulder Press	15	15	15	15	15
Oblique Crunch	15	15	15	15	15
Hyperextension	15	15	15	15	15

CARDIOVASCULAR EXERCISE

Fast Walk	30	30	30	30	30

168

Combat Fat!

ADVANCED WORKOUT

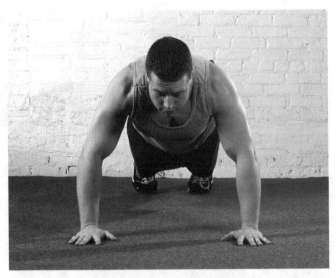

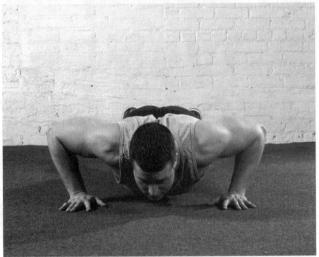

Push-up

Regular push-ups are challenging and are a great upper body exercise that firms and strengthens your arms, shoulders and chest. Lay on the ground with your hands placed flat next to your chest. Push yourself up by straightening your arms and while keeping your back straight.

170

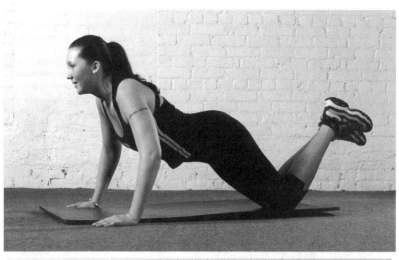

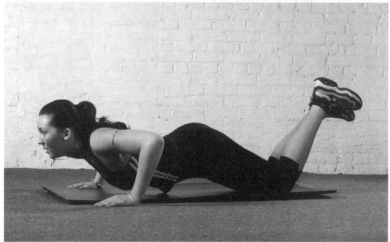

Push-up on Knees

Start on your hands and knees, lower your chest close to the floor, then push away from the floor, straightening your arms.

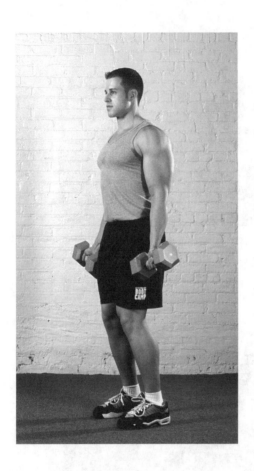 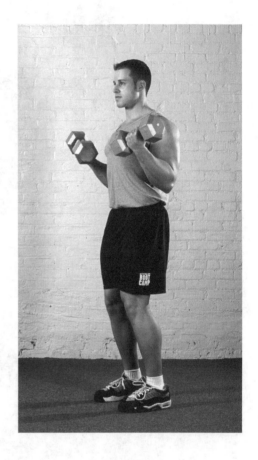

Biceps Curl

Start with a weight in each hand and your elbows next to your sides. Keep your back straight and knees slightly bent. Lift your hands to your chest by bending your arms, bringing the weights up in a controlled motion.

172

w.combat-fat.com www.combat-fat.com www.combat-fat.com www.combat-fat.com www.combat-fat.

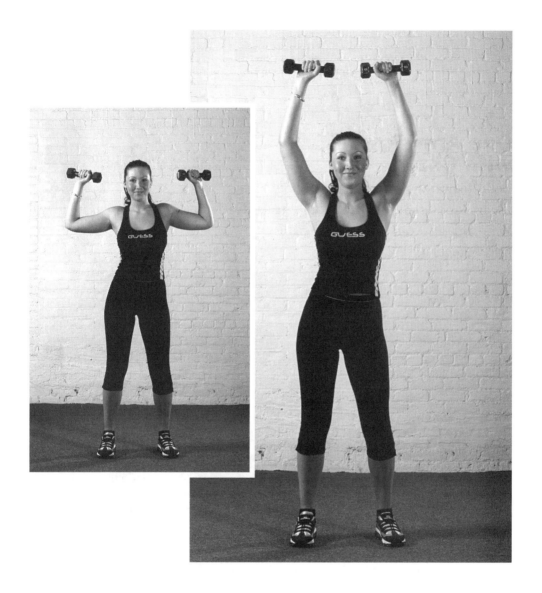

Standing Shoulder Press

Place your feet about shoulder-width apart, keeping your knees slightly bent. Exhale as you push the weights over your head. Slowly lower them to shoulder height and repeat.

173

One Arm Row with Chair

Bend forward at the waist, holding the back of a chair with the your left arm and let your right arm hang fully extended.

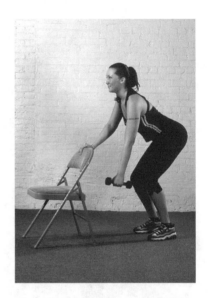

Pull the weight up to your waist. Keep your trunk stable throughout the exercise. Switch arms and repeat.

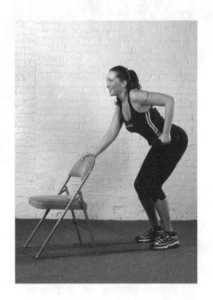

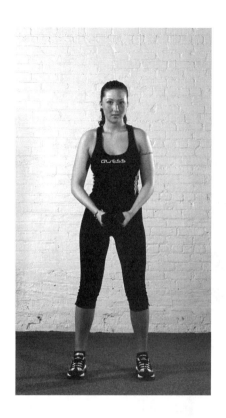 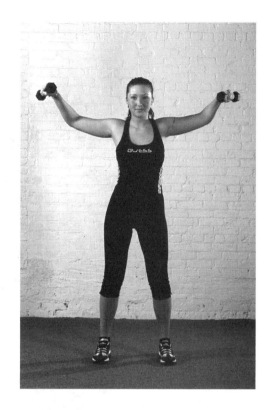

Lateral Raise

Stand up with your knees bent and your back straight and your arms at either side. Hold a dumbbell in each hand. Lift the weights directly out to the sides of your body until they reach the level of your cheeks. Hold the weights there for a one-second count. Slowly descend, lowering the dumbbells in a controlled fashion back to the starting point.

175

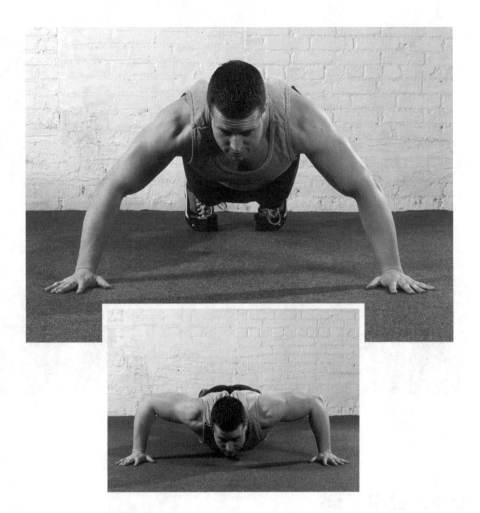

Wide Push-ups

Wide hand placement isolates your chest muscles more intensely. Place your hands wider than shoulder width apart to perform this push-up variation.

176

.combat-fat.com www.combat-fat.com www.combat-fat.com www.combat-fat.com www.combat-fat.

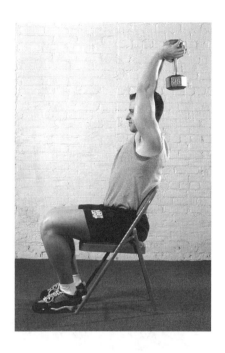 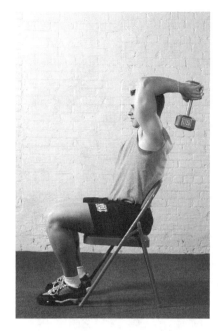

Triceps Extension

Sit at the end of a flat exercise bench in a stable chair and place your feet on the floor about shoulder-width apart. During this exercise, keep your elbows pointing up toward the ceiling at all times. Raise the weight over your head as you straighten your arms. Slowly bend your elbows and lower the dumbbell down toward your neck area. Make sure not to go too low, because trying to raise the dumbbell from this position can put stress on your elbow joints. Slowly raise the dumbbell back to the starting position. Hold this position for a one-second count and while you contract the muscles of your triceps.

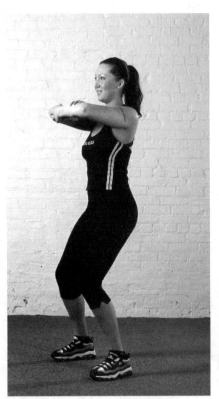 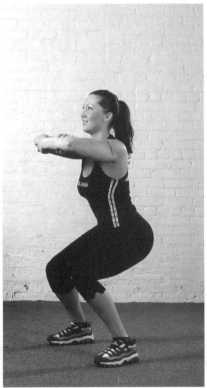

Parallel Squat

This exercise is excellent for toning your legs and buttocks. Make sure you perform it with feet flat, trying not to go onto your toes when squatting, which places too much pressure on your knees and ankles. For the same reason, be careful not to bend your knees greater than 90 degrees. In order to keep your feet flat, spread your legs a little wider than shoulder width apart.

178

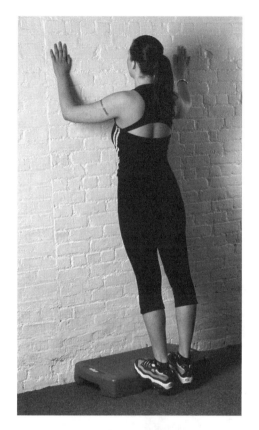
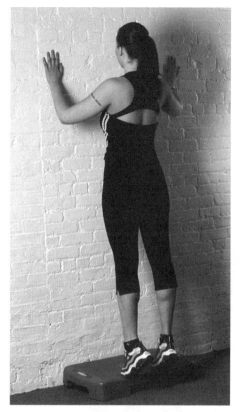

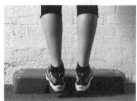
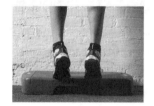

Intermediate Heel Raise

Stand on a platform and lean slightly against a wall for balance. Lift your-self up onto your toes and back down slowly. (You can also perform this exercise one leg at a time for an even greater challenge.) This exercises tones your calves and strengthens your ankles.

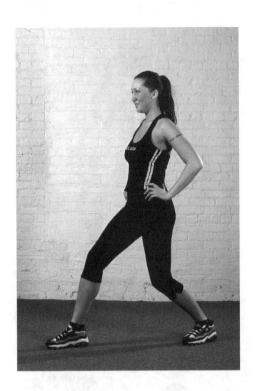 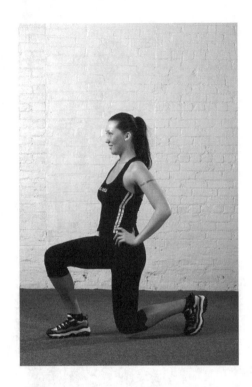

Stationary Lunge

The lunge builds lower body strength and flexibility. It intensifies the work-load on the forward leg and challenges your balance. Keeping your chest high and your back straight, take a long step forward and drop your back knee toward the ground. Do not bend more than 90 degrees, and keep your knee directly over your ankle as shown.

Complete the set amount of repetitions with the right foot before stepping out with the left. (You might notice that the exercise looks like you're doing a one legged squat; this is what you want.)

If you have serious knee problems even the stationary lunge may be too strenuous for you. If so, repeat the squat exercise instead of the lunge.

180

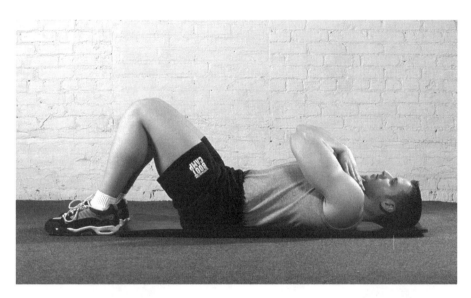

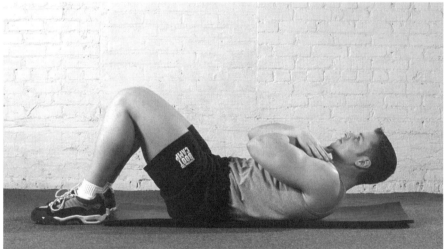

Crunch with Hold

Perform a basic crunch by lifting your shoulders off the floor. When you reach the lifted position, hold it for 5 seconds before lowering.

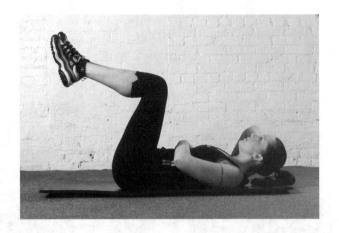

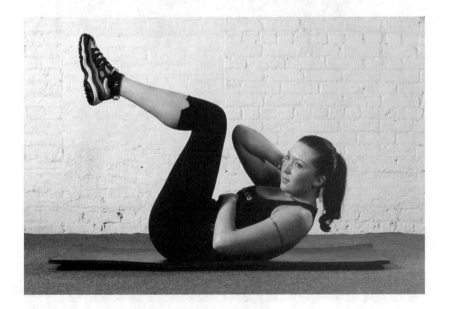

Advanced Oblique Crunch

Lay on your back with your knees bent and your feet in the air. Lift your chest off the floor, twisting to bring your right elbow to your left knee. Switch sides and repeat.

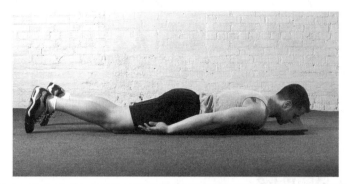

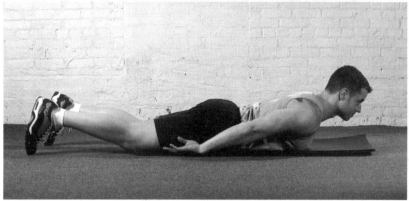

Hyperextension

Lay face down, with your hands resting at the sides of your body. Slowly raise your torso about 2-3 inches from the ground, and hold for a 3-second count. This small movement helps strengthen your lower back. When you begin raising your torso, slightly arch your upper back, shoulders and head. If you encounter any type of pain during this exercise, STOP! Also, do not fatigue your lower back muscles. Stop when you start to feel a tight sensation.

Combat Fat! Advanced Workout Week #1

DAY #1 DAY #2 DAY #3 DAY #4 DAY #5

FLEXIBILITY

All stretches should be performed daily.

RESISTANCE EXERCISES

	Day 1	Day 2	Day 3	Day 4	Day 5
Push-up	10		10		10
Biceps Curl		10		10	
Shoulder Press	10		10		10
One-Arm Row	10		10		10
Lateral Raise	10		10		10
Wide Push-ups	10		10		10
Triceps Extension		10		10	
Parallel Squat		10		10	
Heel Raise		10		10	
Lunges		10		10	
Crunch with Hold	10		10		10
Advanced Oblique Crunch	10		10		10
Hyperextension	10		10		10

CARDIOVASCULAR EXERCISE

	Day 1	Day 2	Day 3	Day 4	Day 5
Run/Jog or Bike	30	30	30	30	30

A NOTE ON SELECTING THE PROPER AMOUNT OF WEIGHT FOR RESISTANCE TRAINING
The weight you select for each exercise depends on the amount of repetitions you need to do for a particular set. If you need to do between 10-12 repetitions for one set, pick a weight where you fail (the point at which completing another repetition becomes impossible) between 10-12 reps. This takes a bit of practice but after a while you will become extremely accurate when it comes to choosing the correct weight for a particular repetition range. If you pick a weight that allows you to do more than 12 repetitions, you'll need to increase the amount of weight being lifted. If you reach failure before hitting the tenth rep, you'll need to decrease the amount of weight being lifted.

184

Combat Fat! Advanced Workout Week #2

DAY #1   DAY #2   DAY #3   DAY #4   DAY #5

FLEXIBILITY

All stretches should be performed daily.

RESISTANCE EXERCISES

	DAY #1	DAY #2	DAY #3	DAY #4	DAY #5
Push-up	12		12		12
Biceps Curl		12		12	
Shoulder Press	12		12		12
One-Arm Row	12		12		12
Lateral Raise	12		12		12
Wide Push-ups	12		12		12
Triceps Extension		12		12	
Parallel Squat		12		12	
Heel Raise		12		12	
Lunges		12		12	
Crunch with Hold	12		12		12
Advanced Oblique Crunch	12		12		12
Hyperextension	12		12		12

CARDIOVASCULAR EXERCISE

	DAY #1	DAY #2	DAY #3	DAY #4	DAY #5
Run/Jog or Bike	30	30	30	30	30

185

Combat Fat! Advanced Workout Week #3

FLEXIBILITY

All stretches should be performed daily.

RESISTANCE EXERCISES

	DAY #1	DAY #2	DAY #3	DAY #4	DAY #5
Push-up	12		12		12
Biceps Curl		12		12	
Shoulder Press	12		12		12
One-Arm Row	12		12		12
Lateral Raise	12		12		12
Wide Push-ups	12		12		12
Triceps Extension		12		12	
Parallel Squat		12		12	
Heel Raise		12		12	
Lunges		12		12	
Crunch with Hold	12		12		12
Advanced Oblique Crunch	12		12		12
Hyperextension	12		12		12

CARDIOVASCULAR EXERCISE

	DAY #1	DAY #2	DAY #3	DAY #4	DAY #5
Run/Jog or Bike	30	30	30	30	30

186

Combat Fat! Advanced Workout Week #4

FLEXIBILITY

All stretches should be performed daily.

RESISTANCE EXERCISES

	DAY #1	DAY #2	DAY #3	DAY #4	DAY #5
Push-up	12		12		12
Biceps Curl		12		12	
Shoulder Press	12		12		12
One-Arm Row	12		12		12
Lateral Raise	12		12		12
Wide Push-ups	12		12		12
Triceps Extension		12		12	
Parallel Squat		12		12	
Heel Raise		12		12	
Lunges		12		12	
Crunch with Hold	12		12		12
Advanced Oblique Crunch	12		12		12
Hyperextension	12		12		12

CARDIOVASCULAR EXERCISE

	DAY #1	DAY #2	DAY #3	DAY #4	DAY #5
Run/Jog or Bike	30	30	30	30	30

187

Combat Fat! Advanced Workout Week #5

FLEXIBILITY

All stretches should be performed daily.

RESISTANCE EXERCISES

Exercise	DAY #1	DAY #2	DAY #3	DAY #4	DAY #5
Push-up	15		15		15
Biceps Curl		15		15	
Shoulder Press	15		15		15
One-Arm Row	15		15		15
Lateral Raise	15		15		15
Wide Push-ups	15		15		15
Triceps Extension		15		15	
Parallel Squat		15		15	
Heel Raise		15		15	
Lunges		15		15	
Crunch with Hold	15		15		15
Advanced Oblique Crunch	15		15		15
Hyperextension	15		15		15

CARDIOVASCULAR EXERCISE

Exercise	DAY #1	DAY #2	DAY #3	DAY #4	DAY #5
Run/Jog or Bike	35	35	35	35	35

188

Combat Fat! Advanced Workout Week #6

	DAY #1	DAY #2	DAY #3	DAY #4	DAY #5

FLEXIBILITY

All stretches should be performed daily.

RESISTANCE EXERCISES

	DAY #1	DAY #2	DAY #3	DAY #4	DAY #5
Push-up	15		15		15
Biceps Curl		15		15	
Shoulder Press	15		15		15
One-Arm Row	15		15		15
Lateral Raise	15		15		15
Wide Push-ups	15		15		15
Triceps Extension		15		15	
Parallel Squat		15		15	
Heel Raise		15		15	
Lunges		15		15	
Crunch with Hold	15		15		15
Advanced Oblique Crunch	15		15		15
Hyperextension	15		15		15

CARDIOVASCULAR EXERCISE

	DAY #1	DAY #2	DAY #3	DAY #4	DAY #5
Run/Jog or Bike	35	35	35	35	35

189

Combat Fat! Advanced Workout Week #7

| DAY #1 | DAY #2 | DAY #3 | DAY #4 | DAY #5 |

FLEXIBILITY

All stretches should be performed daily.

RESISTANCE EXERCISES

	DAY #1	DAY #2	DAY #3	DAY #4	DAY #5
Push-up	2/10		2/10		2/10
Biceps Curl		2/10		2/10	
Shoulder Press	2/10		2/10		2/10
One-Arm Row	2/10		2/10		2/10
Lateral Raise	2/10		2/10		2/10
Wide Push-ups	2/10		2/10		2/10
Triceps Extension		2/10		2/10	
Parallel Squat		2/10		2/10	
Heel Raise		2/10		2/10	
Lunges		2/10		2/10	
Crunch with Hold	2/10		2/10		2/10
Advanced Oblique Crunch	2/10		2/10		2/10
Hyperextension	2/10		2/10		2/10

CARDIOVASCULAR EXERCISE

	DAY #1	DAY #2	DAY #3	DAY #4	DAY #5
Run/Jog or Bike	35	35	35	35	35

190

Combat Fat! Advanced Workout Week #8

DAY #1 DAY #2 DAY #3 DAY #4 DAY #5

FLEXIBILITY

All stretches should be performed daily.

RESISTANCE EXERCISES

	DAY #1	DAY #2	DAY #3	DAY #4	DAY #5
Push-up	2/10		2/10		2/10
Biceps Curl		2/10		2/10	
Shoulder Press	2/10		2/10		2/10
One-Arm Row	2/10		2/10		2/10
Lateral Raise	2/10		2/10		2/10
Wide Push-ups	2/10		2/10		2/10
Triceps Extension		2/10		2/10	
Parallel Squat		2/10		2/10	
Heel Raise		2/10		2/10	
Lunges		2/10		2/10	
Crunch with Hold	2/10		2/10		2/10
Advanced Oblique Crunch	2/10		2/10		2/10
Hyperextension	2/10		2/10		2/10

CARDIOVASCULAR EXERCISE

	DAY #1	DAY #2	DAY #3	DAY #4	DAY #5
Run/Jog or Bike	35	35	35	35	35

Combat Fat!

ELITE
WORKOUT

Chest Press

The dumbbell bench press develops tight and toned chest muscles. Begin by taking hold of two dumbbells and lay back on a flat bench or the floor. Position the dumbbells to the outside of your chest, keeping the elbows wide throughout the exercise movement and the forearms perpendicular to the floor.

Press the dumbbells up toward the ceiling. Hold for a 2 second count. Slowly lower the weights.

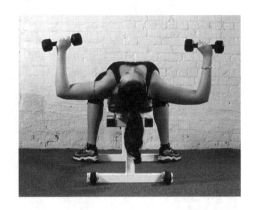

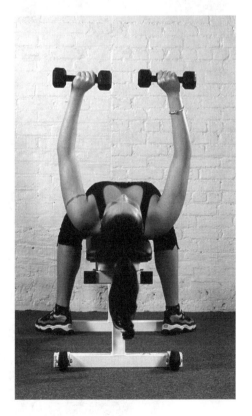

Lat Pulldown

The lat pulldown exercise is a great exercise for building the muscles of the mid and upper back region.

Position the thigh support so that your thighs fit snug under the pads with your feet flat on the floor. Choose your desired weight and take a grip equal to 1 1/2 times your shoulder length. Pull the bar down towards your collar bone, maintaining good posture.

At the bottom of the movement, squeeze your back muscles for a count of 1 second with. Slowly return to the start position.

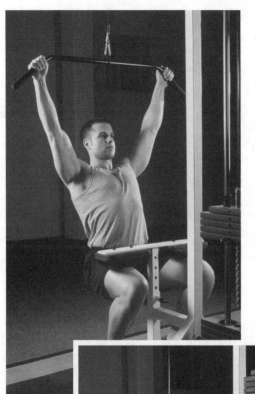

194

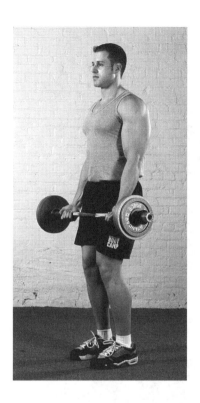 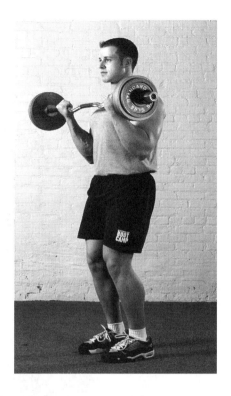

Barbell Curl

Hold the barbell at arm's length, resting it against your upper thighs. Curl the barbell in a semicircular motion until your forearms touch your biceps. Make sure to keep your upper arms close to your sides when curling. Slowly return to the starting position. Do not move your torso back and forth to help lift the weight. This not only takes tension off the biceps, but it can also hurt your lower back.

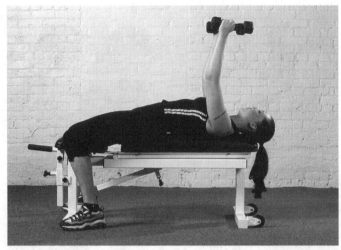

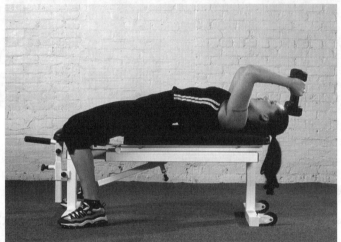

Dumbbell Triceps Lying

Hold a dumbbell in each hand, keeping the portion of your arms from the shoulder to elbow locked in place. Allow the portion of your arms from the elbow to the hands to slowly bend down towards your shoulders. Just before touching the dumbbells to the shoulders, return your arms to the start position.

196

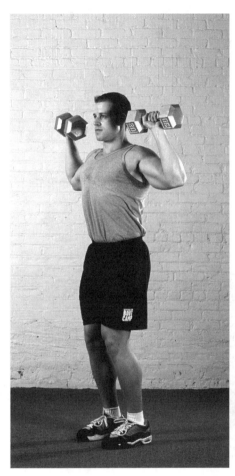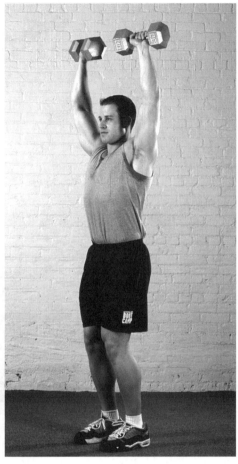

Shoulder Press

Place your feet shoulder width apart, keeping your knees slightly bent to help reduce strain on your lower back. Exhale as you push the weights over your head. In a smooth and controlled motion, slowly lower the weights to the starting position.

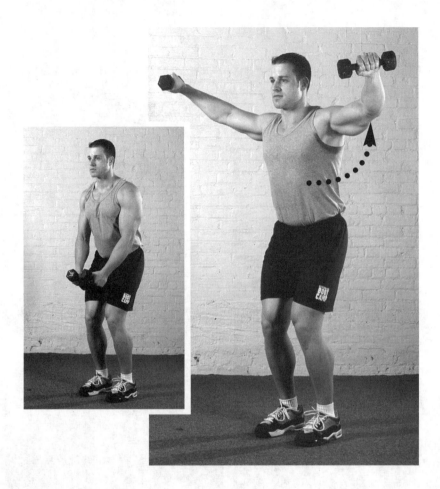

Lat Raise

This is a great exercise for building shoulder and upper arm strength. Start by holding a dumbbell in each hand and, with a slight bend at the elbow, your arms positioned at each side of your body. Your palms should be facing the sides of your body at all times.

Lift the weights directly out to the sides of your body until they reach the level of your cheeks. Hold the weights in this position for a one-second count. Lower the dumbbells in a controlled fashion to the starting position.

198

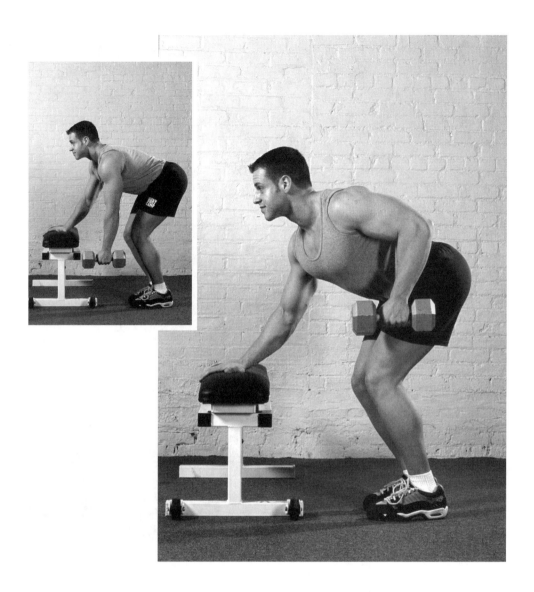

One Arm Row

Bend forward at the waist, taking hold of the back of a chair with your right arm. Holding a weight, let your left arm hang fully extended. Pull the weight back to waist height. Keep your trunk stable throughout the full range of motion. Switch arms and repeat.

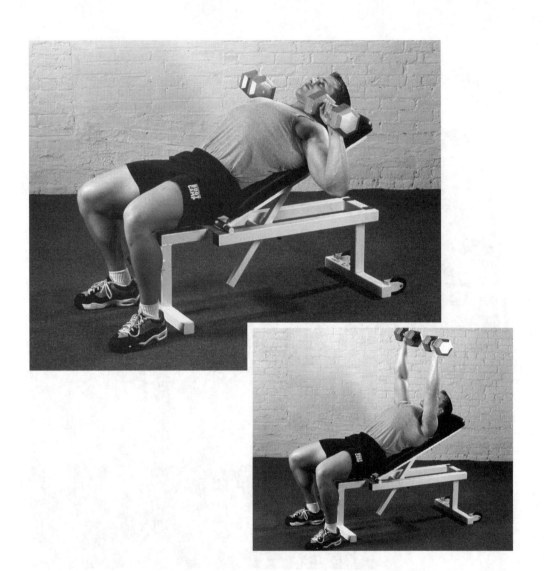

Incline Dumbbell Press

This is a great exercise for developing the muscles of the upper chest. Press the dumbbells up toward the ceiling and squeeze your chest muscles. Begin slowly lowering the weight back to the start position.

200

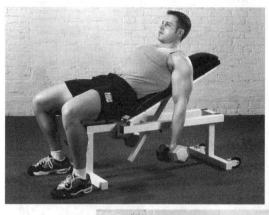

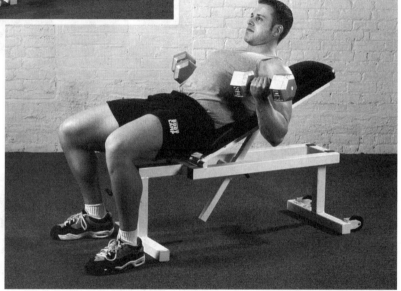

Incline Dumbbell Curl

Set the bench incline to a 45 degree angle. Lean all the way back into the bench and let the dumbbells hang at your sides, making sure that the palms of your hands are facing forwards throughout the motion. Curl the dumbbells, bringing them to the front of your shoulders. Squeeze your biceps and hold the position for a count of two. Slowly and smoothly lower the dumbbells back to the start position.

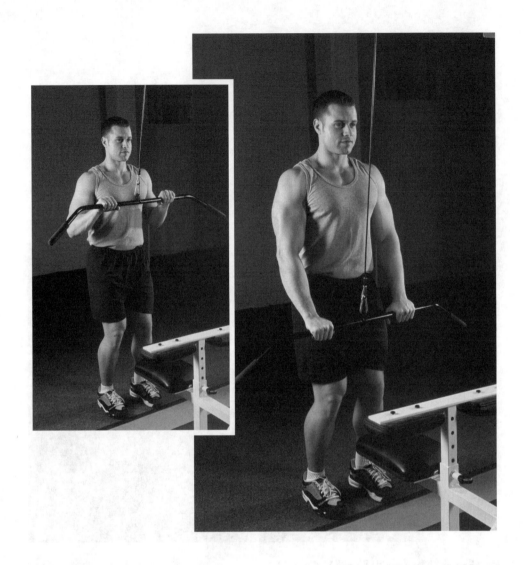

Triceps Pushdown

Start with the bar about chest high and with your arms tucked against your sides. Push down until you reach full extension, but do not lock your elbows. Squeeze your triceps muscles as hard as you can. Slowly allow the bar to return to the starting position, maintaining good posture throughout.

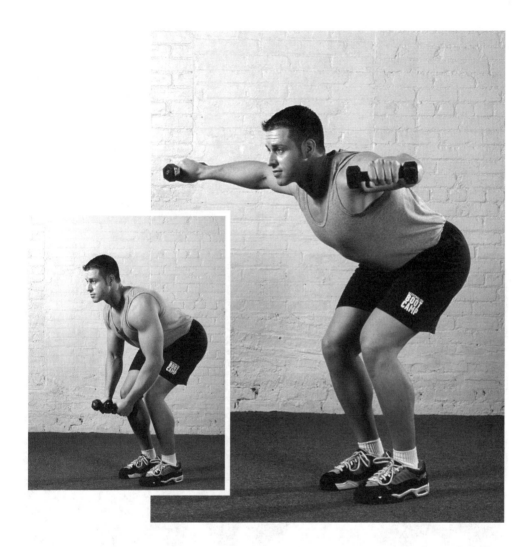

Reverse Fly

Stand with your feet shoulder width apart, slightly bending your knees. Bend forward at the waist while keeping your back flat. Keep your stomach tight. Let the weights hang by your toes, then lift them outward so they are parallel to your shoulders. Concentrate on squeezing your shoulder blades together. Slowly return to the start position.

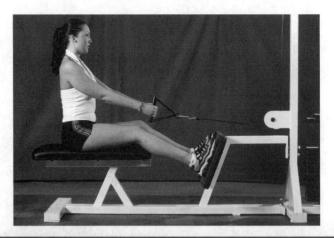

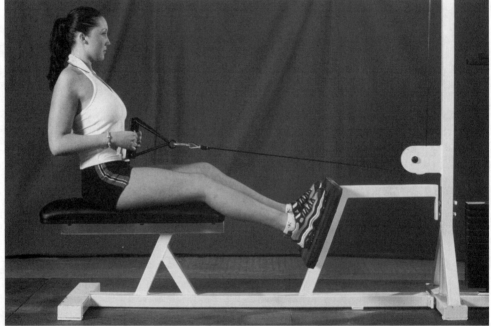

Seated Row

Make sure to keep your legs slightly bent. Lean forward at the hips and grab the row bar. Slowly sit up straight and hold that position. With your back straight and chest forward, slowly pull the handle back toward your mid-section. Concentrate the motion on your upper back and shoulder muscles rather than your arms. Keep your elbows close to your side. Hold for a two-second count and return to the starting position.

204

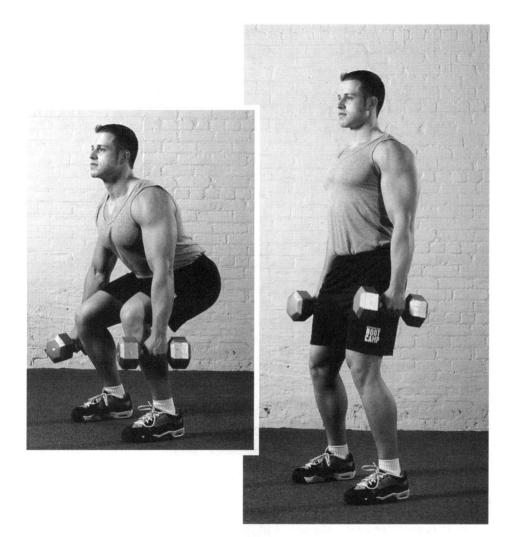

Squats with Dumbbells

Perform this exercise with your feet flat, trying not to go onto your toes when squatting, which places too much pressure on your knees and ankles. For the same reason, be careful not to bend your knees greater than 90 degrees. In order to keep your feet flat, spread your legs a little wider than shoulder width apart.

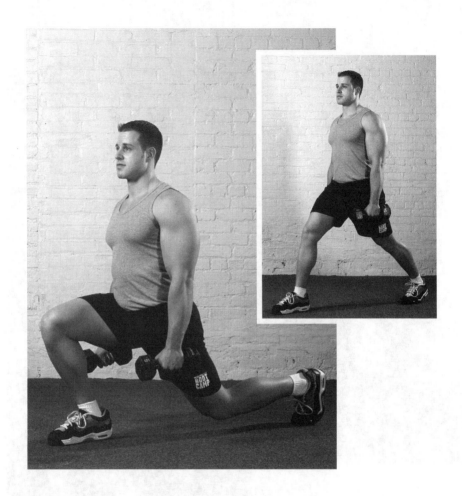

Lunges with Dumbbells

Perform this exercise like a standard lunge, only this time perform the exercise with dumbbells.

If you have knee problems, even the stationary lunge may be too strenuous for you. If so, repeat the squat exercise instead of the lunge.

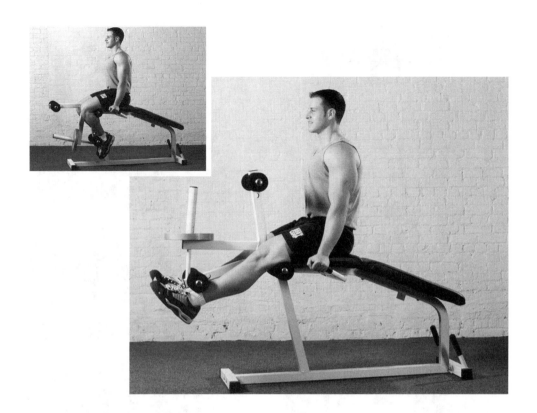

Leg Extension

Sit upright with the back of your knees pressed flush against the front of the seat. Adjust the shin roller pad so it rests against the lowest point of your shin. Slowly raise the weight by lifting the roller pad with your shins. As you reach the point of full extension contract the muscles on the front of your thighs. Slowly return to the beginning of the movement.

207

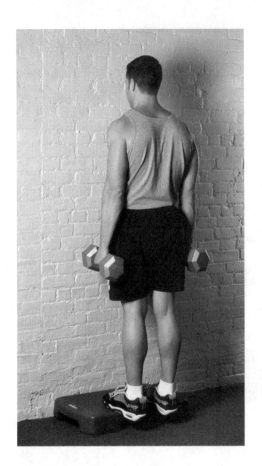 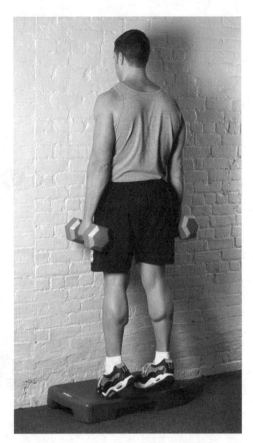

Heel Raise with Dumbbells

Holding a weight in each hand, stand on a platform and lean slightly against a wall for balance. Lift yourself up onto your toes and back down slowly. (You can also perform this exercise one leg at a time for an even greater challenge.) This exercises tones your calves and strengthens your ankles.

208

.combat-fat.com www.combat-fat.com www.combat-fat.com www.combat-fat.com www.combat-fat.

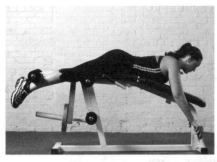

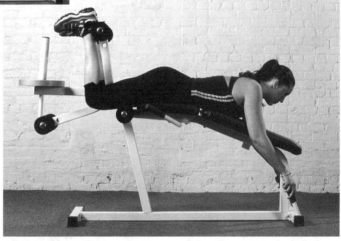

Lying Leg Curl

Begin lifting the weight by pulling with your heels to your butt, while focusing on isolating the muscles on the back of your thighs. When you've reached the top position, hold that position for a two-second count. As you descend downward, do so in a slow, controlled movement.

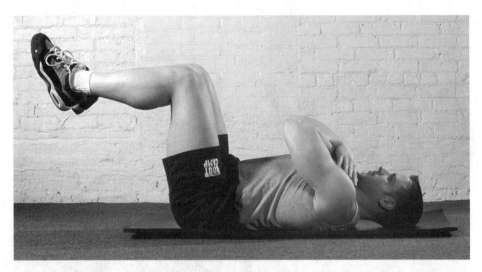

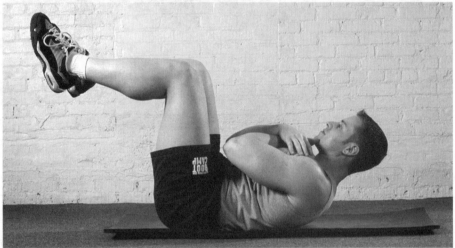

Crunch

Lay on your back with your feet and knees in the air. Cross your hands over your chest and lift your shoulders off the ground, squeezing your abdominal muscles. Hold the "up" position for two-seconds, then slowly release to the starting position.

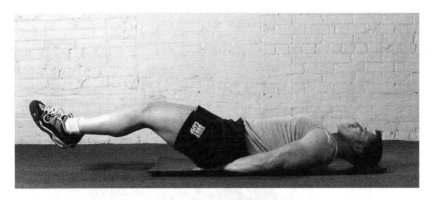

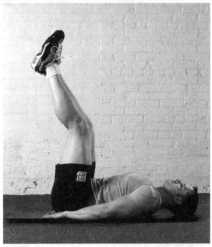

Leg Lift

Start with your feet about six inches from the floor. Place your hands underneath your buttocks for lower back support, keeping them there for the entire duration of the exercise. With your head relaxed, your feet slightly separated from one another and your knees bent as shown above, raise your legs approximately 20 inches off the floor. Use your abdominal muscles exclusively. Use smooth, controlled motions. Return to the start position.

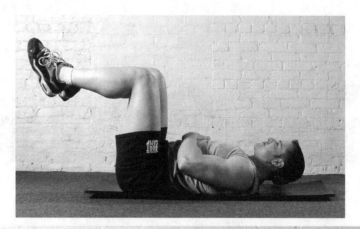

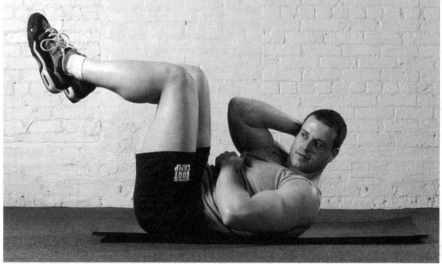

Advanced Oblique Crunch

Lay on your back with your knees bent and your feet in the air. Lift your chest off the floor, twisting to bring your right elbow to your left knee. Switch sides and repeat.

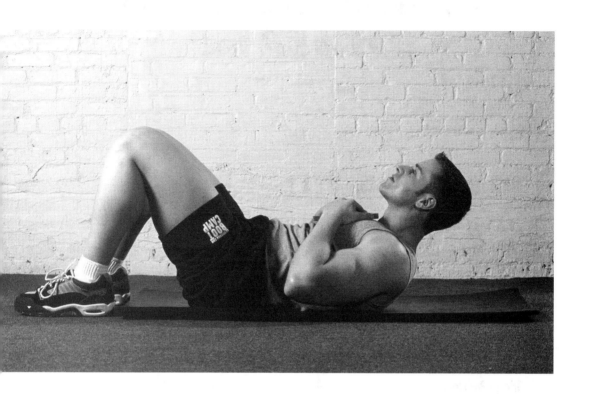

Weighted Crunch

With a weight plate, medicine ball, or dumbbell on your chest, lay on your back with your feet and knees in the air. Lift your shoulders off the ground, squeezing your abdominal muscles. Hold the "up" position for two-seconds, then slowly release to the starting position.

Combat Fat! Elite Workout Week #1

FLEXIBILITY

All stretches should be performed daily.

RESISTANCE EXERCISES

Exercise	Day #1	Day #2	Day #3	Day #4	Day #5
Chest Press	3/10		3/10		3/10
Lat Pulldown	3/10		3/10		3/10
Barbell Curl		3/10		3/10	
Dumbbell Triceps Lying		3/10		3/10	
Shoulder Press	3/10		3/10		3/10
Lat Raise	3/10		3/10		3/10
One-Arm Row	3/10		3/10		3/10
Incline Dumbbell Press	3/10		3/10		3/10
Incline Dumbbell Curl		3/10		3/10	
Triceps Pushdown		3/10		3/10	
Reverse Fly	3/10		3/10		3/10
Seated Row	3/10		3/10		3/10
Squats w/Dumbbells		3/10		3/10	
Lunges		3/10		3/10	
Leg Extension		3/10		3/10	
Heel Raise		3/10		3/10	
Lying Leg Curl		3/10		3/10	
Crunch	3/10		3/10		3/10
Leg Lift					
Oblique Crunch	3/10		3/10		3/10
Weighted Crunch	3/10		3/10		3/10

CARDIOVASCULAR EXERCISE

Exercise	Day #1	Day #2	Day #3	Day #4	Day #5
Run, Bike, Stair Climb	35	35	35	35	35

214

Combat Fat! Elite Workout Week #2

FLEXIBILITY

All stretches should be performed daily.

RESISTANCE EXERCISES

	Day #1	Day #2	Day #3	Day #4	Day #5
Chest Press	3/10		3/10		3/10
Lat Pulldown	3/10		3/10		3/10
Barbell Curl		3/10		3/10	
Dumbbell Triceps Lying		3/10		3/10	
Shoulder Press	3/10		3/10		3/10
Lat Raise	3/10		3/10		3/10
One-Arm Row	3/10		3/10		3/10
Incline Dumbbell Press	3/10		3/10		3/10
Incline Dumbbell Curl		3/10		3/10	
Triceps Pushdown		3/10		3/10	
Reverse Fly	3/10		3/10		3/10
Seated Row	3/10		3/10		3/10
Squats w/Dumbbells		3/10		3/10	
Lunges		3/10		3/10	
Leg Extension		3/10		/10	
Heel Raise		3/10		3/10	
Lying Leg Curl		3/10		3/10	
Crunch	3/10		3/10		3/10
Leg Lift					
Oblique Crunch	3/10		3/10		3/10
Weighted Crunch	3/10		3/10		3/10

CARDIOVASCULAR EXERCISE

	Day #1	Day #2	Day #3	Day #4	Day #5
Run, Bike, Stair Climb	40	40	40	40	40

215

Combat Fat! Elite Workout Week #3

DAY #1   **DAY #2**   **DAY #3**   **DAY #4**   **DAY #5**

FLEXIBILITY

All stretches should be performed daily.

RESISTANCE EXERCISES

Exercise	Day #1	Day #2	Day #3	Day #4	Day #5
Chest Press	3/12		3/12		3/12
Lat Pulldown	3/12		3/12		3/12
Barbell Curl		3/10		3/10	
Dumbbell Triceps Lying		3/10		3/10	
Shoulder Press	3/10		3/10		3/10
Lat Raise	3/10		3/10		3/10
One-Arm Row	3/12		3/12		3/12
Incline Dumbbell Press	3/12		3/12		3/12
Incline Dumbbell Curl		3/10		3/10	
Triceps Pushdown		3/12		3/12	
Reverse Fly	3/12		3/12		3/12
Seated Row	3/12		3/12		3/12
Squats w/Dumbbells		3/12		3/12	
Lunges		3/12		3/12	
Leg Extension		3/10		3/10	
Heel Raise		3/10		3/10	
Lying Leg Curl		3/10		3/10	
Crunch	3/12		3/12		3/2
Leg Lift					
Oblique Crunch	3/10		3/10		3/10
Weighted Crunch	3/10		3/10		3/10

CARDIOVASCULAR EXERCISE

Exercise	Day #1	Day #2	Day #3	Day #4	Day #5
Run, Bike, Stair Climb	40	40	40	40	40

216

FLEXIBILITY

All stretches should be performed daily.

RESISTANCE EXERCISES

Exercise	Day #1	Day #2	Day #3	Day #4	Day #5
Chest Press	3/10		3/12		3/12
Lat Pulldown	3/12		3/12		3/12
Barbell Curl		3/12		3/12	
Dumbbell Triceps Lying		3/12		3/12	
Shoulder Press	3/12		3/12		3/12
Lat Raise	3/12		3/12		3/12
One-Arm Row	3/12		3/12		3/12
Incline Dumbbell Press	3/12		3/12		3/12
Incline Dumbbell Curl		3/12		3/12	
Triceps Pushdown		3/12		3/12	
Reverse Fly	3/12		3/12		3/12
Seated Row	3/12		3/12		3/12
Squats w/Dumbbells		3/12		3/12	
Lunges		3/12		3/12	
Leg Extension		3/12		3/12	
Heel Raise		3/12		3/12	
Lying Leg Curl		3/12		3/12	
Crunch	3/12		3/12		3/12
Leg Lift					
Oblique Crunch	3/12		3/12		3/12
Weighted Crunch	3/10		3/10		3/10

CARDIOVASCULAR EXERCISE

Exercise	Day #1	Day #2	Day #3	Day #4	Day #5
Run, Bike, Stair Climb	35	35	35	35	35

Combat Fat! Elite Workout Week #5

FLEXIBILITY

All stretches should be performed daily.

RESISTANCE EXERCISES

Exercise	Day #1	Day #2	Day #3	Day #4	Day #5
Chest Press	3/13		3/13		3/13
Lat Pulldown	3/13		3/13		3/13
Barbell Curl		3/13		3/13	
Dumbbell Triceps Lying		3/13		3/13	
Shoulder Press	3/13		3/13		3/13
Lat Raise	3/13		3/13		3/13
One-Arm Row	3/13		3/13		3/13
Incline Dumbbell Press	3/13		3/13		3/13
Incline Dumbbell Curl		3/13		3/13	
Triceps Pushdown		3/13		3/13	
Reverse Fly	3/13		3/13		3/13
Seated Row	3/13		3/13		3/13
Squats w/Dumbbells		3/13		3/13	
Lunges		3/13		3/13	
Leg Extension		3/13		3/13	
Heel Raise		3/13		3/13	
Lying Leg Curl		3/13		3/13	
Crunch	3/13		3/13		3/13
Leg Lift					
Oblique Crunch	3/13		3/13		3/13
Weighted Crunch	3/10		3/10		3/10

CARDIOVASCULAR EXERCISE

Exercise	Day #1	Day #2	Day #3	Day #4	Day #5
Run, Bike, Stair Climb	40	40	40	40	40

Combat Fat! Elite Workout Week #6

FLEXIBILITY

All stretches should be performed daily.

RESISTANCE EXERCISES

Exercise	Day #1	Day #2	Day #3	Day #4	Day #5
Chest Press	3/15		3/15		3/15
Lat Pulldown	3/15		3/5		3/15
Barbell Curl		3/13		3/13	
Dumbbell Triceps Lying		3/13		3/13	
Shoulder Press	3/15		3/15		3/15
Lat Raise	3/15		3/15		3/15
One-Arm Row	3/15		3/15		3/15
Incline Dumbbell Press	3/15		3/15		3/15
Incline Dumbbell Curl		3/13		3/13	
Triceps Pushdown		3/13		3/13	
Reverse Fly	3/15		3/15		3/15
Seated Row	3/15		3/15		3/15
Squats w/Dumbbells		3/15		3/15	
Lunges		3/15		3/15	
Leg Extension		3/15		3/15	
Heel Raise		3/15		3/15	
Lying Leg Curl		3/15		3/15	
Crunch	3/15		3/15		3/15
Leg Lift					
Oblique Crunch	3/15		3/15		3/15
Weighted Crunch	3/10		3/10		3/10

CARDIOVASCULAR EXERCISE

Exercise	Day #1	Day #2	Day #3	Day #4	Day #5
Run, Bike, Stair Climb	40	40	40	40	40

219

Combat Fat! Elite Workout Week #7

| DAY #1 | DAY #2 | DAY #3 | DAY #4 | DAY #5 |

FLEXIBILITY

All stretches should be performed daily.

RESISTANCE EXERCISES

Exercise	Day #1	Day #2	Day #3	Day #4	Day #5
Chest Press	3/15		3/15		3/15
Lat Pulldown	3/15		3/15		3/15
Barbell Curl		3/15		3/15	
Dumbbell Triceps Lying		3/15		3/15	
Shoulder Press	3/15		3/15		3/15
Lat Raise	3/15		3/15		3/15
One-Arm Row	3/15		3/15		3/15
Incline Dumbbell Press	3/15		3/15		3/15
Incline Dumbbell Curl		3/15		3/15	
Triceps Pushdown		3/15		3/15	
Reverse Fly	3/15		3/15		3/15
Seated Row	3/15		3/15		3/15
Squats w/Dumbbells		3/15		3/15	
Lunges		3/15		3/15	
Leg Extension		3/15		3/15	
Heel Raise		3/15		3/15	
Lying Leg Curl		3/15		3/15	
Crunch	3/15		3/15		3/15
Leg Lift					
Oblique Crunch	3/15		3/15		3/15
Weighted Crunch	3/15		3/15		3/15

CARDIOVASCULAR EXERCISE

Exercise	Day #1	Day #2	Day #3	Day #4	Day #5
Run, Bike, Stair Climb	40	40	40	40	40

220

Combat Fat! Elite Workout Week #8

DAY #1 DAY #2 DAY #3 DAY #4 DAY #5

FLEXIBILITY

All stretches should be performed daily.

RESISTANCE EXERCISES

Exercise	Day #1	Day #2	Day #3	Day #4	Day #5
Chest Press	3/15		3/15		3/15
Lat Pulldown	3/15		3/15		3/15
Barbell Curl		3/15		3/15	
Dumbbell Triceps Lying		3/15		3/15	
Shoulder Press	3/15		3/15		3/15
Lat Raise	3/15		3/15		3/15
One-Arm Row	3/15		3/15		3/15
Incline Dumbbell Press	3/15		3/15		3/15
Incline Dumbbell Curl		3/15		3/15	
Triceps Pushdown		3/15		3/15	
Reverse Fly	3/15		3/15		3/15
Seated Row	3/15		3/15		3/15
Squats w/Dumbbells		3/15		3/15	
Lunges		3/15		3/15	
Leg Extension		3/15		3/15	
Heel Raise		3/15		3/15	
Lying Leg Curl		3/15		3/15	
Crunch	3/15		3/15		3/15
Leg Lift					
Oblique Crunch	3/15		3/15		3/15
Weighted Crunch	3/15		3/15		3/15

CARDIOVASCULAR EXERCISE

Exercise	Day #1	Day #2	Day #3	Day #4	Day #5
Run, Bike, Stair Climb	45	45	45	45	45

221

8
Combat Fat!
Motivation

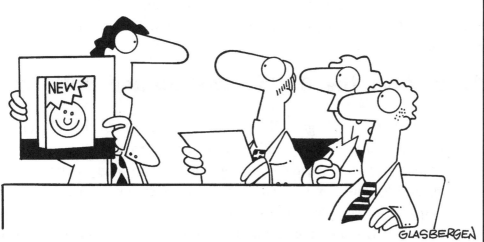

© 1998 Randy Glasbergen.

"Our new product has no fat, no cholesterol,
no calories, no sugar, no salt and no preservatives.
The box is empty, but it has exactly what everyone wants!"

Preparing Yourself Mentally for Change

In this age of yoga and east-meets-west philosophy we all acknowledge the connection between our minds and bodies. One has a strong and powerful influence over the other. This is especially true in the area of weight loss and exercise. To change your body, you need to change your mindset. If you focus solely on your diet or on your workout program, or even on both of these combined without addressing the mental aspects of making a lifestyle change, you most likely will not be able to maintain your results in the long-term. And what good is it to lose fat just for a few months only to gain it right back? That only makes us feel unsuccessful and helpless.

Scientific evidence shows that addressing the psychology behind why we eat what we eat is vital to ensuring long-term results. Experts recognize that the only way to successfully change diet and exercise behavior is to take a three-pronged approach that incorporates nutritional counseling, an exercise program, and a psychological component. We will deal with this third component now.

1. Achieve the Right Attitude and Beliefs

Above all, you must undergo a change in your attitude and beliefs. You need to look inward to understand fully why you may overeat or not exercise. You may be an emotional eater—you eat when you are angry, depressed, or even happy. Or, you may be a lazy eater—you just grab whatever food is easiest and closest to you without thinking about its nutritional value. Likewise, you may not exercise because you fear you aren't good at it, or you may find it too painful and unenjoyable, or feel that you don't have the time for exercise. Whatever attitudes or beliefs are sabotaging your attempts at fitness, it is crucial that you get to the root of them. This is the only way that you can be sure that you are getting to the core of your unhealthy habits. Exercising and dieting alone without addressing these issues is like bandaging a wound without ever really fixing it. You need to include the mental component as well to achieve true success.

224

As a first step, determine your current attitude toward weight loss by answering the following questions:

- How many times have you tried to lose weight or exercise regularly?

- How long have the successful results from these attempts lasted?

- Why do you think you gained back the weight or stopped exercising?

- How did you feel when you gained back the weight?

- Do you feel confident that you will be able to achieve your weight loss goals?

- Do you believe that you can commit to change your lifestyle so that your results will last a lifetime?

The answers to these questions provide you with a baseline assessment of your current attitudes and beliefs about weight loss. They make clear exactly how you feel—right now—about your prior weight loss attempts. If you answered that you felt like a failure when you gained back the weight, you need to acknowledge that feeling (because our feelings are valid and need to be recognized) but then set it aside. Your past attempts, are simply that—something in your past.

They are not failures. Think about your weight loss process not as a series of failed attempts but as a multi-landscaped journey that naturally involves ups, downs and plateaus. During your journey, there will be times when you may slip or fall; that's not the time to give up and turn back. Rather it's the time to get up again and keep climbing to a more fit leaner, healthier life. Believe that you can reach your weight loss goals and you will.

Having the confidence and ability to avoid temptation when faced with difficult situations is called self-efficacy by social researchers. They have found it is vital to have a high level of self-efficacy or belief in your ability to succeed. Remember the childrens' story about the little engine that could? Just like the engine in the story, you need to believe in your abilities, even when the going gets tough.

Researchers also have found that all behavioral change (whether to stop smoking, drinking or to lose weight) is a process that unfolds over time.

2. Recognize that Change Occurs in Stages

One of the most respected and widely followed theories of behavior change is *The Stages of Change* developed by the researchers Prochaska and DiClemente. *They propose that all changes in behavior involved cycling through a series of stages of readiness to change.* Prochaska and DiClemente developed their model after studying smokers who were trying to kick the habit. They found that smokers changed their behavior (stopped smoking) through a series of stages. At each stage, there were certain mental and behavioral strategies that helped them to effectively move on to the next stage in the process.

The stage model has been adapted to cover a wide range of health behaviors including obesity and sedentary lifestyles. *It states that change involves progressing through the following five stages: precontemplation, contemplation, preparation, action and maintenance.* Determine which stage you are in with regard to fat loss:

Precontemplation
In precontemplation you do not plan to change your behavior; in fact, you are very unmotivated and resistant to change. Since you are reading this book you probably are not in this first

226

stage. Congratulations! You are at the very least in the next stage, contemplation.

Contemplation

Contemplation is the stage in which you are seriously thinking about changing your behavior. In fact you intend to change within the next six months. You want to lose the weight and start exercising because you believe it is important for your health and quality of life. But, you also may be plagued by negative thoughts at this stage. You are worried about how much time you'll need to spend exercising, how much it will cost to join a gym or whether you will be able to follow a healthy eating plan. If you are at this stage, we will help you to address your concerns so that you can move on to the next stage. Now is also the time to consider some unexpected sources of resistance to change.

Examining Some Hidden Obstacles to Getting Started

Do you feel helpless and hopeless about your prospects? Maybe this is an attitude that blocks you in many aspects of your life. Learn to activate the virtue of hope

Do you secretly like being fat? Maybe you identify with celebrities who were fat, like Alfred Hitchcock. It makes you feel important, like you stand out in a crowd.

Are you afraid to be thin? Maybe your heaviness has served as a protection against being hurt by others. Learn to handle emotional issues psychologically instead of physically, the way they should be handled.

Do you think you will lose friends by getting in shape? Chances are that you will become a model for many of your friends who are also struggling with too much fat.

Are you afraid of being too attractive if you're thin, maybe even too sexually attractive? If you are, give thought to what conflicts exist here and try to resolve them in a healthier way.

Will being thin mean you will have to throw out your favorite clothes and buy new ones? Sorry, but that's part of the price you'll have to pay for being a healthier, happier human being.

Do you think the "real you" will disappear? The fun-loving overweight person who loved to carouse and was the butt of other's jokes will become so thin that you will not be visible any more, and the space you used to take up will be occupied by someone else? You will find that you can live with that and that the genuine light of your real personality will shine even more brightly.

Preparation

In preparation you are ready to take action in the immediate future. You are highly motivated and have a positive attitude about your ability to change. You are ready to go! If you are in this stage, you are ready to set your goals and begin the Combat Fat! body fat measuring, eating and exercising plan.

228

Action

The action stage is characterized by actually being immersed in your behavior change. Once you begin the Combat Fat! program, you will be in action. During this stage we recommend that you continue to use techniques such as self-monitoring, stimulus control and social support to ensure your continued success in the maintenance stage.

Maintenance

Maintenance means that you have reached your goals and now are working to prevent a relapse (which we will call a temporary slip-up). We will show you some proven strategies to avoid a relapse, such as avoiding high risk situations, as well as how you can cope with a slip-up if it should occur—without derailing from the Combat Fat! program.

3. Stay Motivated

The more motivation you have when undergoing any type of behavior change, the greater your chances for long-term success. Keeping your motivation high is essential in all of the stages of change—from contemplation to maintenance. So how can you get and—more importantly—remain motivated?

Believe that You Can Win the Fat Battle

First, really understand that being over-fat is not merely a matter of aesthetics. It is in fact a very serious condition that greatly jeopardizes both your physical and emotional health. Scientists don't fully understand why some people are more prone to getting fat than others. Most likely genetics and your basic metabolism play a role, but eating and exercising habits definitely have been established as key factors in maintaining a healthy body composition. Knowing this is empowering. After all, if it were simply a matter of some "fat" gene we've inherited, then we'd have about as much luck changing our bodies as we do the color of our eyes. In truth, obesity is directly related to our nutritional habits and our level of activity—the better our diets and the greater our activity the less fat we carry. This gives us tremendous control over the composition of our bodies. As long as we set realistic and attainable goals, following a scientific-based program for reducing body fat, such as Combat Fat!, will lead to success!

Believing in your ability to change involves several ancillary beliefs.

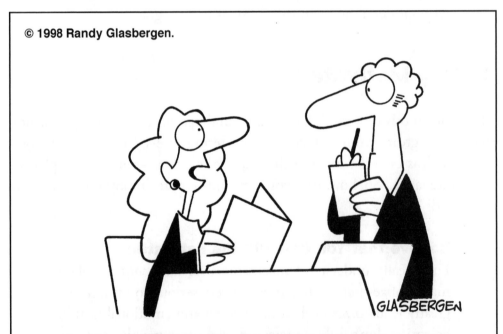

© 1998 Randy Glasbergen.

GLASBERGEN

"I'm going to order a broiled skinless chicken breast, but I want you to bring me lasagna and garlic bread by mistake."

Have faith in yourself and in the power of your commitment to change. When you have a bad day, turn to that which makes you spiritually strong, whether it be prayer, meditation or listening to music.

Overcome inertia. Second in difficulty to maintaining a healthy lifestyle in the long term is being able to overcome inertia in the first place. You've already made it to the point where you are interested in changing. Now the next big step is to make the actual plan to change (and then of course to do it).

Recognize that some long held habits and beliefs on your part are about to be tossed away. For example you may be used to rewarding yourself for getting through your hectic day with a pint of ice cream every night. This habit will need to be changed to a more healthy reward. It will not be easy, but it is necessary.

Accept that there will be some physical and mental pain as you begin to change your behavior. We are creatures of habit and any habit—good or bad—is hard to break. We are trying to cultivate healthy habits here. As pain is a natural part of any growth process, expect some here, and know that it will not last forever.

Overcome Your Barriers

Second, you need to overcome the barriers (or excuses) to engaging in and successfully achieving and maintaining your fat-loss goals. While each person's barriers may differ, there are some common ones that we can address here.

Excuse #1: I have no time to exercise

It is a bit ironic that although we live in an advanced technological society with a myriad of objects designed to save us time that most of us feel more pressed for time than our parents or grandparents did. It seems like the more time gadgets save us, the more we pile on our plates. Here are some tips to successfully carve out time (at least 30 minutes each day) for physical activity.

Wake up a half hour earlier and get your workout in before you begin your busy day. This way, no matter what unexpected setbacks the day throws at you, you will have done your workout. (Working out in the morning also is a great energy booster. You'll find that you'll have more energy throughout the day and feel great.)

For one week consciously take note and record time spent on non-essential sedentary tasks, with an eye to using this time more productively. For example, how many hours do you spend watching television, reading magazines, or eating meals? Try to carve a few minutes off of each of these activities until you have accumulated at least a half hour for your exercise.

Incorporate activity into your daily life activities. Walk to work or to the store instead of automatically getting into your car. We are so programmed to drive everywhere that we often drive when we could easily have walked. Ask yourself when was the last time you took the stairs instead of an escalator?

232

Realize that exercise is not an extraneous activity. It is as essential to your health as eating and sleeping. Even if it means you need to cut back on some other activities, you need to truly think of it as becoming a part of your life, not apart from it.

Excuse #2: I hate to exercise

Most people who hate to exercise don't give themselves enough time to become adept at their activity. They quit before their bodies have been able to adapt to the new demands of their workout. You need to accept that exercise for most of us is difficult and can be uncomfortable initially—especially if you have been sedentary for a long time. This discomfort is normal and to be expected. Rest assured, if you stick with your exercise plan it will get more and more comfortable and actually enjoyable. Best of all, you'll feel the sense of satisfaction that comes with having faced up to a challenge.

There are any number of activities you can do to increase your fitness. The options are endless and include power walking, swimming, running, working on your garden, etc. Choose one that appeals to you—not to your friends. Just because "everybody else loves kickboxing" if it doesn't appeal to you, don't force yourself to do it—because chances are you won't be able to go the full-distance.

Human beings were made to move. We have legs, and arms and core muscles that propel us forward. It is unnatural for us to be so sedentary. Incorporate any kind of movement into your life. Go dancing. Bowl.

233

Whatever it is, as long as you're body is in motion; you're doing good things for your health and fitness.

If you are doing regular fitness exercises, choose your place of exercise to maximize your motivation. The privacy of your home. A small gym with a trainer where there are few, if any, others there at the time. A glitzy club, complete with music, beautiful and not-so-beautiful people, where you have a plethora of machines to use and they serve free bagels (which of course you turn down). As one experienced trainer observed: "The most powerful factor that encourages exercise is distance—how close your gym is from your home or office."

Excuse #3: A special diet and exercise plan? Sounds expensive and boring.

Many diets require that you purchase specific foods or pay a fee. This is a big barrier for those of us with financial considerations. The Combat Fat! program enables you to fold a healthy eating plan into your life without additional cost. All of the recipes included in Part III use ingredients commonly found in homes. In addition, our exercise programs can be done at home as easily as at a gym, making it unnecessary for you to join a local heath club (although joining a gym can provide social support and added incentive to remain active).

Far from boring, the Combat Fat! eating plan is full of nutritious healthy and delicious meals that you and your whole family will enjoy. This is not a diet, there are no gimmicks, no shakes that you have to drink

234

morning, noon and night. It is a livable plan for healthy eating. Essentially you will learn how to eat the way that lean people eat all the time.

Excuse #4 : Based on past experience, I don't really believe I'll be successful

As we've said before, changing a behavior is far from easy. If it were, there would be no need for this book. However you now know that behavior change occurs in stages, and that it is normal to have many so called failed attempts before achieving success. This does not mean you will never be successful. You will, but you need to be in a state of readiness to change your unhealthy lifestyle habits. Just as a smoker can only cease smoking when he or she is truly ready, you will only be able to effectively change your eating and exercising habit when you are determined to and believe in your capacity for change.

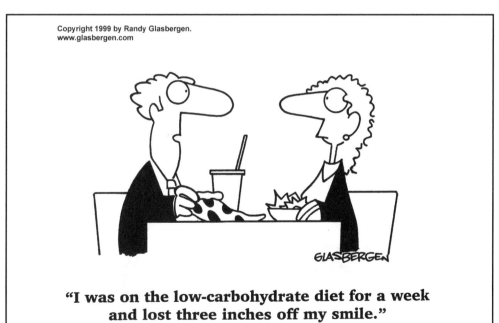

"I was on the low-carbohydrate diet for a week and lost three inches off my smile."

Strategies for Success

The following eight strategies have been widely studied and used by cognitive-behavioral therapists to help thousands of people. Some of them are directly related to the way you think or the attitudes and beliefs you may need to overcome (this is the cognitive aspect of change). Others have to do with changing habits and engaging in behaviors that support change, such as monitoring your progress in the areas of diet, fitness and body fat measurement.

Set Realistic and Attainable Goals

Honestly assess where you are and where you can reasonably expect to be. You may want to look like a fashion model or athlete, but how realistic is that? Truth is that while we can do much to change our appearance, we are limited to an extent by the blueprint of our genes. This does not mean that we are destined at birth to be either fat or lean, but it does mean that we shouldn't expect to look exactly like someone who is petite with small bones, if our bone structure is large and we are tall.

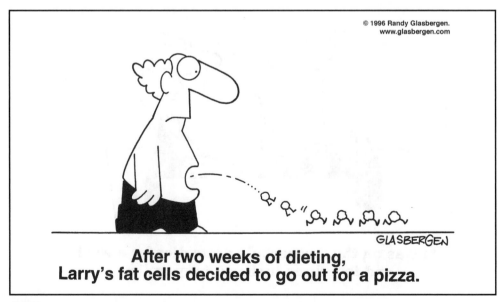

After two weeks of dieting,
Larry's fat cells decided to go out for a pizza.

You need to focus on being the healthiest and most fit you can be given your own biological and social circumstances. For instance, if you are someone with plenty of free time to devote to exercise, you probably will become leaner in a shorter amount of time than if you are crunched for time. You need to take several factors into consideration when determining your fat-loss goals, and make them attainable both in the short and long-term. In Part II of the Combat Fat! Program we help you to determine your body fat percentage goals.

As far as time frame goes, government experts consider a 10 percent reduction in weight loss over a six-month period reasonable. Remember, this program deals with fat loss not weight loss per se (although, of course the two are related), so the time frame may be a bit different.

Self-Monitor Your Eating Habits and Physical Activity

Self-monitoring is a key technique you can use to support your behavior change. In self-monitoring you record data daily related to your diet and exercise behaviors, which will provide personal insight into your behaviors. You can then use this data to help you to set your goals, monitor your progress, and as a way to inform you of those situations or emotional states which place you at risk for overeating or under-exercising.   Here's how self-monitoring works:

For Your Diet

Each day record the amount and types food that you eat in your dietary log (see Appendix). You must include every single food eaten. This will give you a sense of what you are eating. In addition, next to each entry record the time and place that you ate the food, your level of hunger, and what you were feeling—your emotional state—before and after eating. Note too what was going on at the time: were you with other people, watching television, talking on the telephone, under stress?

SAMPLE DAILY DIETARY LOG					
Monday	**Time:**	**Time:**	**Time:**	**Time:**	**Time:**
Food Eaten					
Place					
Situation					
Happenings					
Level of Hunger					
Emotional State Before Eating					
Emotional State After Eating					

For Your Exercise Plan

Record your fitness behavior in a fitness log (see appendix). The log should include a record of the frequency, intensity and type of physical activity you engaged in as well as when and where you exercised, and how you felt before and after your workout. If you do not workout on a particular day, indicate why and how you felt that day.

SAMPLE FITNESS LOG							
Week of:	Monday	Tuesday	Wednesday	Thursday	Friday	Saturday	Sunday
Activity							
Duration							
Time							
Place							
Emotional State Before Workout							
Emotional State After Workout							

Your Body Fat Log

Since the Combat Fat! program focuses on achieving and maintaining a healthy body composition—in other words, a healthy percentage of body fat—it will be helpful for you to monitor your level of body fat on a weekly basis. And put your scales in storage. In his article in *Essential Psychopharmacology* on the management of eating disorders, Dr. Zerbe describes the folly and futility of taking one's weight over and over again and being emotionally affected by the numbers; when he sees patient who are obsessed with such behavior, he shows them how simply moving the scale from one part of the room to another can change the results by several pounds. Remember: it's fat we're after, not pounds!

Part II of this book discusses body fat in detail and how you will be able to measure your level of fat easily at home using the skin fold caliper you can order for free with this book. Refer to your body fat log to determine how well you are doing in reaching your ultimate body fat goals. Body fat measurements should be taken before exercising and at the same time each week (first thing in the morning is a great time).

MONITOR YOUR PROGRESS								
	Week 1	Week 2	Week 3	Week 4	Week 5	Week 6	Week 7	Week 8
Body Fat Percentage								

Learn to Manage Stress

Does devouring a pint of chocolate chip ice cream soothe your nerves at the end of a bad day at work? It comes as no surprise that many of us eat poorly when we are under stress. It's easy to do. After all, from the time we are small children food has been used to comfort us. But you can learn to effectively manage stressful situations without going straight to the fridge or nearest fast food restaurant. Here are some strategies you can use:

Change Your Perspective: If you perceive an event as threatening or stressful, you will experience it as such. Try to cast a negative event in a positive light. For example, if your boss has been putting you under a lot of pressure by giving you too many assignments, consider that it may be because he or she holds you in great esteem. Recognizing this can give you the confidence to address the situation with your boss and work out a more manageable work schedule. Also, make a mental note that whatever stress you currently feel will dissipate. It will not last forever so you don't need to obsess over it. Think about something else.

240

Problem Solve: Sometimes we eat as a way of avoiding a problem or stress. Instead of thinking about possible solutions to our problem, we eat French-fries. When faced with a stressful problem, try to come up with workable solutions. You may need to do research to gather information, or ask friends and family for advice. Do something active and creative about your situation and you'll be less likely to eat your way out of it.

Regulate your Emotions: Sometimes it is important to express our feelings in order to release stress. It is important to vent your feelings and not keep them bottled up inside. This doesn't mean you need to tell off everybody who annoys you, but you do need to express in a constructive way when someone has hurt or angered you.

Try Relaxation Techniques: There are many ways to actively relax your body. When you are in a state of relaxation you are less likely to feel stressed. A few methods follow.

- *Deep Breathing.* When you feel anxious or stressed out take a few minutes to do deep breathing. Focus your mind on your breath as you inhale extra slowly (to a count of four) and then exhale to a count of four. Make sure you start your breath from your diaphragm instead of from your chest. Imagine that with each inhale you are blowing up a large balloon.

241

- *Yoga.* Regularly doing a stretch and breathing-based type of exercise, such as yoga, can help you put stress into perspective and leave you relaxed and refreshed.

- *Massage.* Treat yourself to a body massage to release tension from your body and mind

- *Meditate.* Take ten minutes out of each day, preferably first thing in the morning, to sit quietly and meditate. Clear your mind, focus on your breathing and commit to preserving a healthy, positive perspective throughout the day.

Become More Resilient. Resilience is made up of the physical, mental, emotional, and situational requirements to enable you to deal effectively with any kind of stress or change, and to rebound when you have experienced one of life's many set-backs. Eating healthier and exercising regularly enhance your resilience. Surrounding yourself with positive people and enjoying your work and working relationships is part of it. To learn more about how to become resilience you might want to read Dr. Frederic Flach's outstanding book on the subject: *Resilience: The Power to Bounce Back When the Going Gets Tough.*

Develop Problem Solving Skills

We already mentioned that problem solving is one way to manage stress. You also can use it to correct your own personal problem areas related to eating and physical activity. First, of course, you need to identify these problem areas, which may be revealed to you through the information in your dietary and fitness logs. Once you've identified these problem areas, you can brainstorm possible solutions, select one, and then plan and implement a healthier alternative. You can do this alone, or preferably, with the assistance of a lifestyle management professional or counselor.

For example, let's say that your logs indicate a pattern of eating unhealthily when you feel rushed or are pressed for time. You just grab the quickest food, often a high-fat, calorie-laden one. In addition, you notice that the first thing you forgo when time-pressed is your workout. It is clear that you need to do something to better manage your time, so you brainstorm several solutions from getting up earlier, to going to bed later to cutting some dispensable activities from your day. You decide the easiest thing you can do is get up an hour earlier each day and this is the solution you implement.

Control the Stimuli That Make You Want to Eat

You're not even thinking about eating when you walk by the fast food hamburger restaurant down the block from your home. Suddenly the scent of fries and a cheeseburger wafts through the air. Before you know it you're on line ordering a super combo. So much for the healthy chicken salad that you had planned on eating for dinner! Maybe you should have walked home on the other side of the street!

One of the key ways that you can prevent over-eating or eating poorly is to control stimuli that encourage eating. This is also known as avoiding high-risk situations, meaning those situations in which you are most likely to eat poorly. Of course, sometimes they're unavoidable, and you'll just have to sweat them out. Everyone's high-risk situations differ, which is why you need to maintain your dietary log. It will provide valuable clues into those stimuli that have the strongest effect on you. The following are some common stimulus control strategies to reduce the temptation to eat:

- *Shop carefully.* Read labels when you shop, making sure that you choose the healthiest, freshest foods.

- *Keep unhealthy high-calorie foods out of your house.* If there aren't any cookies in the cupboard, you'll be more apt to choose a piece of fruit as a snack.
- *Never shop when hungry.* Shop on a full stomach and you'll be less likely to pile your cart high with food.

- *Avoid the dessert aisle at the supermarket.*

- *Eat a healthy snack before you go to a party or picnic where over-eating is likely to occur and you'll be less tempted to over-indulge.*

- *Bring your lunch to work every day and you won't be tempted by less healthy choices.*

- *Avoid going to restaurants that have the high-calorie foods that tempt you most.*

- *Control portions.* Portion out your foods on your plate and then put the rest of the food away. Do not leave it out to tempt you to take seconds.

Successfully Handle Temporary Setbacks
A key area related to problem solving is learning how to effectively deal with a relapse. Relapses are very common in all

behavior change. In weight loss in particular, people often find they hit plateaus or walls that they can't get over and this can sometimes lead to frustration and resumption of old habits. Unfortunately, the relapse can then spiral downward to you feeling that you have absolutely failed.

Just because you over-indulge one day, or miss exercising for a couple of days does not mean that you have failed in your attempts to change your behavior. You simply have experienced a lapse, a temporary setback or slip-up, which can in fact be turned into a positive! How? Think of the lapse as a valuable learning experience: ask yourself "What did I earn from this setback?" Maybe you've discovered a new food-specific cue, or emotional stimulus. If for say, you have a lapse in response to problems you are having with your spouse, it may indicate the need for some professional help or counseling. Remember too, that once the lapse is over, it's over and you are right back on track again.

In *Relapse Prevention* (Guilford Press, 1985), author G. Alan Marlatt, offers the following strategies you can use when you lapse.

- *Listen to what the lapse is telling you.* It is a signal that you need to address the situation.
- *Remain calm.* You may feel guilty initially. This is normal and will pass. Be careful not to punish yourself. Lapses happen.

- *Renew your commitment to changing your behavior.*

- *Review the events, feelings, etc. that led up to your lapse and try to identify warning signals.*

245

Try Contingency Management: Planned Rewards

Contingency management involves rewarding yourself for positive specific actions, such as increasing time spent walking or reducing consumption of specific foods. Rewards can be monetary, social, or personal—something that will help you to maintain your motivation and commitment throughout all the stage of change. For example, when you are in the action stage midway to your fat-loss goal you might treat yourself to a new outfit, a day at a spa, or simply a long, relaxing massage.

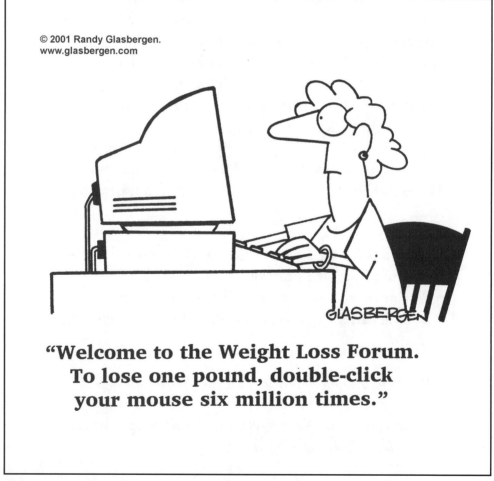

© 2001 Randy Glasbergen.
www.glasbergen.com

"Welcome to the Weight Loss Forum.
To lose one pound, double-click
your mouse six million times."

Build a Support Network

A strong system of social support is very helpful during the action and maintenance stages. Turn to family and friends for positive reinforcement and motivation. Of course the key is to surround yourself with people who are truly supportive, encouraging and positive about your behavior change. Try to get your whole family on a healthy eating and exercising plan; it will provide support for your efforts and will be doing everyone a service. Steer clear of people who are negative or critical about your efforts. Negativity is the last thing you need right now.

Another option is to join a weight loss support group—either in person or online. And, working out with a buddy is an effective way to keep stay motivated, as is hiring a personal trainer.

With Combat Fat! you have access to the interactive support of health and fitness experts as well as people like you who are on the program. Simply go to www.combat-fat.com to benefit from the support of others in the program.

Appendix
Combat Fat!
Goodies

Combat Fat! Website Information
Blank Menu Creation Forms
Body Fat Measurement Tables
Progress Charts
Free Body Fat Caliper Offer

The Combat Fat! Website
www.combat-fat.com

There is no question that social support networks are essential to succeeding in life. Friends, family, your Church, for example, all can provide meaningful relationships which can help you achieve your life goals and overcome life's obstacles.

The same applies to your health and fitness. There is no need to feel in isolation as you pursue your goal of leading a healthier life through the Combat Fat! program. To this end we have created a virtual community for you to find friends, gain encouragement, share experiences, and help others achieve their goals, too.

Whether you find a virtual partner on the internet, or a have a friend or family member who wants to join in your quest for physical excellence, it sure beats going it alone!

So visit the Combat Fat! website at combat-fat.com and discover millions of Americans who share in your desire to look good and feel good. Let's all do this together and achieve extraordinary results!

Combat Fat! Create Your Own Menu Plan

	BREAKFAST	LUNCH	DINNER	SNACK
MONDAY				
TUESDAY				
WEDNESDAY				
THURSDAY				
FRIDAY				
SATURDAY				
SUNDAY				

251

Combat Fat! Create Your Own Menu Plan

	BREAKFAST	LUNCH	DINNER	SNACK
MONDAY				
TUESDAY				
WEDNESDAY				
THURSDAY				
FRIDAY				
SATURDAY				
SUNDAY				

Combat Fat! Create Your Own Menu Plan

	BREAKFAST	LUNCH	DINNER	SNACK
MONDAY				
TUESDAY				
WEDNESDAY				
THURSDAY				
FRIDAY				
SATURDAY				
SUNDAY				

Combat Fat! Create Your Own Menu Plan

	BREAKFAST	LUNCH	DINNER	SNACK
MONDAY				
TUESDAY				
WEDNESDAY				
THURSDAY				
FRIDAY				
SATURDAY				
SUNDAY				

Combat Fat! Body Fat Tables

AGE	SKINFOLD MEASUREMENT IN MILLIMETERS																
	2-3	4-5	6-7	8-9	10-11	12-13	14-15	16-17	18-19	20-21	22-23	24-25	26-27	28-29	30-31	23-33	34-36
UP TO 20	11.3	13.5	15.7	17.7	19.7	21.5	23.2	24.8	26.3	27.7	29.0	30.2	31.3	32.3	33.1	33.9	34.6
21-25	11.9	14.2	16.3	18.4	20.3	22.1	23.8	25.5	27.0	28.4	29.6	30.8	31.9	32.9	33.8	34.5	35.2
26-30	12.5	14.8	16.9	19.0	20.9	22.7	24.5	26.1	27.6	29.0	30.3	31.5	32.5	33.5	34.4	35.2	35.8
31-35	13.2	15.4	17.6	19.6	21.5	23.4	25.1	26.7	28.2	29.6	30.9	32.1	33.2	34.1	35.0	35.8	36.4
36-40	13.8	16.0	18.2	20.2	22.2	24.0	25.7	27.3	28.8	30.2	31.5	32.7	33.8	34.8	35.6	36.4	37.0
41-45	14.4	16.7	18.8	20.8	22.8	24.6	26.3	27.9	29.4	30.8	32.1	33.3	34.4	35.4	36.3	37.0	37.7
46-50	15.0	17.3	19.4	21.5	23.4	25.2	26.9	28.6	30.1	31.5	32.8	34.0	35.0	36.0	36.9	37.6	38.3
51-55	15.6	17.9	20.0	22.1	24.0	25.9	27.6	29.2	30.7	32.1	33.4	34.6	35.6	36.6	37.5	38.3	38.9
56 & UP	16.3	18.5	20.7	22.7	24.6	26.5	28.2	29.8	31.3	32.7	34.0	35.2	36.3	37.2	38.1	38.9	39.5
	LEAN			IDEAL			AVERAGE			OVERFAT							

Data provided by Dr. Andrew S. Jackson (University of Houston) and Dr. Michael L. Pollock (University of Florida).

BODY FAT INTERPRETATION CHART FOR MEN

AGE	SKINFOLD MEASUREMENT IN MILLIMETERS																
	2-3	4-5	6-7	8-9	10-11	12-13	14-15	16-17	18-19	20-21	22-23	24-25	26-27	28-29	30-31	32-33	34-36
UP TO 20	2.0	3.9	6.2	8.5	10.5	12.5	14.3	16.0	17.5	18.9	20.2	21.3	22.3	23.1	23.8	24.3	24.9
21-25	2.5	4.9	7.3	9.5	11.6	13.6	15.4	17.0	18.6	20.0	21.2	22.3	23.3	24.2	24.9	25.4	25.8
26-30	3.5	6.0	8.4	10.6	12.7	14.6	16.4	18.1	19.6	21.0	22.3	23.4	24.4	25.2	25.9	26.5	26.9
31-35	.5	7.1	9.4	11.7	13.7	15.7	17.5	19.2	20.7	22.1	23.4	24.5	25.5	26.3	27.0	27.5	28.0
36-40	5.6	8.1	10.5	12.7	14.8	16.8	18.6	20.2	21.8	23.2	24.4	25.6	26.5	27.4	28.1	28.6	29.0
41-45	6.7	9.2	11.5	13.8	15.9	17.8	19.6	21.3	22.8	24.7	25.5	26.6	27.6	28.4	29.1	29.7	30.1
46-50	7.7	10.2	12.6	14.8	16.9	18.9	20.7	22.4	23.9	25.3	26.6	27.7	28.7	29.5	30.2	30.7	31.2
51-55	8.8	11.3	13.7	15.9	18.0	20.0	21.8	23.4	25.0	26.4	27.6	28.7	29.7	30.6	31.2	31.8	32.2
56 & UP	9.9	12.4	14.7	17.0	19.1	21.0	22.8	24.5	26.0	27.4	28.7	29.8	30.8	31.6	32.3	32.9	33.3
	LEAN			IDEAL			AVERAGE			OVERFAT							

Data provided by Dr. Andrew S. Jackson (University of Houston) and Dr. Michael L. Pollock (University of Florida).

COMBAT FAT! BODY FAT LOG

	Week 1	Week 2	Week 3	Week 4	Week 5	Week 6	Week 7	Week 8
Body Fat Percentage								

COMBAT FAT! FITNESS LOG

Week of:	Monday	Tuesday	Wednesday	Thursday	Friday	Saturday	Sunday
Activity							
Duration							
Time							
Place							
Emotional State Before Workout							
Emotional State After Workout							

COMBAT FAT! DIETARY LOG

Monday	Time:	Time:	Time:	Time:	Time:
Food Eaten					
Place					
Situation					
Happenings					
Level of Hunger					
Emotional State Before Eating					
Emotional State After Eating					

FREE FAT CALIPER OFFER!
($19.95 VALUE!)

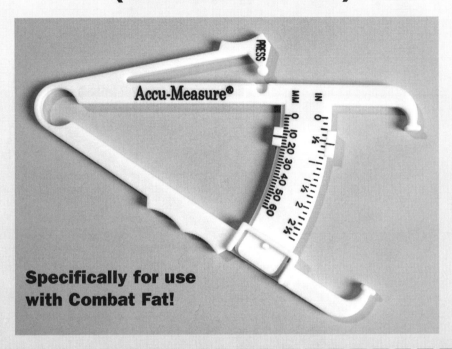

Accu-Measure®

**Specifically for use
with Combat Fat!**